# The Art of Health

AARTI PATEL, N.D.

*For Lukas*

AUTHOR'S NOTE: The information in this book is not intended as a substitute for medical care. *If you have a health problem, consult a medical professional.*

ON CONFIDENTIALITY: The descriptions in *The Art of Health* do not identify individuals. At the heart of naturopathic medicine is confidentiality for each patient, and I have taken careful measures to preserve the privacy of all real persons. All names are fictitious, and all other identifying information has been changed. The people and circumstances portrayed are composite, as in each case represents a mix of individuals whose characteristics and experiences overlapped in nature.

# Contents

*There is no medicine you can take that will replace what you can do for your own health.*

# INTRODUCTION

**What is health?** Toward one extreme, health can conjure up thoughts of a sterile doctor's office or hospital, scary medical words and labels, diagnoses such as diabetes and cancer that sound so final, surgery and open-in-the-back gowns, and strange-sounding pharmaceutical drugs. Visiting the other extreme of alternative health, we picture all things natural, tofu sandwiches, endless vitamins and supplements, yoga and spandex, hugging trees and being one with the earth, visiting a shamanic energy healer, and pouring out our feelings for catharsis. Do either of these camps sound like they describe real health to you?

We often turn to outside sources, both through health care systems and in the mainstream media, to have the ultimate say about our health. We figure that these sources know a whole lot more than we do about how to live a long and healthy life. Yet despite the recommendations, health doesn't always improve like we hope it will. At some point, it's helpful to ask who is the ultimate authority on your health.

Does a doctor know what health is simply because they are a doctor? Does the answer lie inside a bottle of medication or supplements? Perhaps a vegan diet regimen, CrossFit workout, or yoga philosophy? A health website, blog, or magazine? "The Dr. Oz Show," or "The Biggest Loser"? Wait, don't forget that 20/20 piece on health that gave you nightmares. Then there are all those research papers and self-help books out there!

Talk about dizzying amounts of information overload. In reality, health is simpler than that. It can be tempting to search for the answers to health outside yourself. Sure, the sources mentioned above can be useful tools if they're relevant to your health and who you are. But what is the number one and greatest source for living a long and healthy life?

It's YOU. That's right—you have the #1 authority on your health by being the only person who lives in your body, is going through your life, and is facing your own unique challenges. Along the way, you may encounter useful tools in the form of a treatment plan offered by a trusted health care provider, a new diet and exercise routine, or a cool blog post that inspires you to pay more attention to your health. But even these tools will only be useful for the long-term if you develop a real connection with your health, your lifestyle, and what you're going through.

**Health is an art.** Think about all the functions the body performs for us on a daily basis without us being consciously aware of them. The body works in a naturally sophisticated and artful way and if we support what it's already doing for us, we can spark health that best fits who we are as individuals. Each person's life is a unique expression of art too. The best way to practice the art of health is by staying true to who you are throughout it.

I've been practicing naturopathic medicine for six years. In practice, I treat chronic difficult-to-treat conditions in large part by teaching the keys to artful health I talk about here in this book. Though I treat a variety of chronic complaints from insomnia to digestive issues, my specialties are women's health, natural hormone balancing, dermatology, homeopathy, and autoimmune conditions.

Throughout appointments and when coming up with treatment plans, I try and help patients pay more attention to what they're going through and encourage them to take more charge of their health. I know I've done my job when someone feels more confident in how they're approaching health and how they take care of themselves. **When a patient can make connections between their health and lifestyle and see the artfulness inherent in their health care, they have real tools they can use for the long-term.**

My interest in health started from a young age—I wanted to enter the health care field one day, but I also had a vested interest in my own health. I saw from early visits to my pediatrician that doctors' offices only went so far in helping to support health. The main lessons in health seemed to be alive at home, in how I approached my life and how I treated myself as a person. I wondered about the best ways to keep the body and mind healthy, but I also started seeing that no two people's health was alike. Health seemed just as unique as each person, and because of that, strict formulas didn't seem to be the keys to a long and healthy life. What were the keys?

My studies throughout high school and college were heavily focused on science, and pre-medicine specifically, but even in my courses I wasn't seeing what really made people's health tick. There was so much knowledge in my text books, but a key element to health always seemed to be missing. It was the human element, as well as the reality that life and health aren't static or processed inside a laboratory.

No matter how much had been expertly written or researched, these medical concepts didn't seem to explain everything about the human body and how it functioned. My classes taught me what technically and theoretically happened in the body, but it appeared to me from everyday observation that each person's real health extended from unique life experiences and who they were. A topic such as personality, which never showed up in text books, seemed to play a big part in how people approached their health. Over time, something became clearer to me. Health really was an art!

Once I entered naturopathic medical school, I paid close attention for four years to see if I could learn more about how people's health was tied closely to who they were as individuals. I did learn a lot in medical school, but much of it had to do with which treatments were specific to each symptom and condition. The emphasis again seemed to be on the information coming out of a text book, from lab tests, or from a diagnosis. During clinical rotations, however, I got the opportunity to start learning from patients themselves.

I noticed that patients already knew a lot about their health and if just given a chance to discuss what they were going through, they could learn lessons on self care that went far beyond specific treatments or labs. I also saw that it took courage for people to talk about what they were going through, as this practice isn't usually encouraged in our society.

People wanted to learn more about connections in their health, and they wanted to support who they were through health care. I was starting to realize that each individual has a natural ability to support the health of his or her body and lifestyle in a unique and personalized way. In my private practice the last six years, I've gotten to expand even more on what I started learning during those clinical rotations.

Patients often schedule an initial naturopathic appointment with me by describing their main complaint as: "I just haven't been feeling like myself." It takes courage and honesty for someone to admit to themselves that they're feeling this way, let alone tell a health care provider. There are plenty of external and societal pressures to "feel great" and perfect each day despite how you're really feeling. The idea is to fake it until you make it. But you can't fake good health.

When someone says that they don't feel like themselves, they're admitting that they don't want to ignore unbalanced health and everyday chronic symptoms anymore. They want to bring health more into the forefront of life and make it a priority. They want to feel like themselves again and experience increased energy and vitality in life.

Most of all, they start shifting into the mentality that health can't be found in a pill or any "magic" treatment and that only by paying attention to their bodies and how they're feeling, can they make real strides toward getting healthier. This is the philosophy that drew me to natural medicine in the first place, both in my own health and as a profession. Developing a real connection with your body and its health sparks noticeable benefits both in how you look and how you feel.

Picture the following scenario: Waking up tired and without motivation to get up and start the day. Soreness and tightness in the muscles and/or joints, particularly in the neck, upper back, and shoulders. An upset digestive system that brings on sluggishness after meals rather than energy and desire for action. Bloating. Mind fog and difficulty concentrating. Mood swings or irritability. Continuous and heavy fatigue. Cravings for sugary foods or drinks, caffeine, or nicotine to get through the day. Allergies with itching and sneezing.

Wait—there's more. Signs of hormone imbalance. Chronic skin issues such as acne or eczema. Anxiety or depression that lingers all day. Unrelenting stress that seems to keep piling on. Less enjoyment of activities or hobbies that used to be fun. Difficulty maintaining healthy weight, especially around the midsection. Trouble winding down toward the evening. Feeling disconnected from yourself. Trouble falling asleep, or interrupted sleep during the night. Regular under-sleeping or over-sleeping. Dreading the next day. Then, press repeat.

Does that picture feel familiar to you? The

scenario describes common chronic symptoms that many people experience on a daily basis. It shows the **modern day health dilemma,** one that often can't be described by a single medical diagnosis or fixed with one treatment. People don't tend to experience just one or two of these symptoms. They often experience a cluster of them together. Most of the symptoms are related to each other and are riding on a wave of accumulated stress, an overtaxed body and mind, unsupportive lifestyle habits, suppressed thoughts and emotions, unrealistic pressures and expectations on self, unhealthy distractions, and a lack of attention to taking care of the body and mind.

**The truth is, it can become easy to get used to that picture and tolerate it day after day.** To stop questioning it altogether and just accept it as the norm. After all, for most people it's still possible to be successful at work while feeling this way, get through school, attend to family, fulfill daily responsibilities and obligations, meet up with friends, celebrate the holidays, and so on.

We can convince ourselves that life is way too full and busy to do anything about it. Besides, who's asking us to? Thoughts can flood in about the countless list of things that must be done instead. Work is important, and so are bills. There are a bunch of family members and friends to get in touch with, or people that need our help. Family duties, household chores, business matters, finances, a parking ticket, social media, school work,...the list goes on.

The question isn't just *what is health.* It's what is health *to you?* If health is important to you, you can bring more of it into your life. If it remains at the back of the line behind other more important things to do, that's where it'll stay. It's up to you, and it's a natural ability we all have and can take advantage of, to take care of our health and support the innate healing potential of the body.

What makes health a true art form? *You.* You're an artist who holds a paint brush in your hand that creates the unique picture of your health. You naturally have the insight, wisdom, and ability to take care of yourself and bring health into your life using that paint brush. If you want to change the picture to be more in line with who you are and how you'd like to feel in your health, you can do it. And like all art, it takes practice.

Does the chronic symptom picture described above support living life and doing what you want with it? Not really. In truth, unbalanced health blocks life and energy from flowing in the body. We all deal with the challenge of maintaining health in the face of life's challenges. After all, we experience ups and downs and health can't be attained in a separate and perfect bubble outside of that.

That's okay, though. The moment we come to terms with this reality, we can start to pay attention to what's really going on in our bodies throughout life's ever-changing terrain. We can then support our health in a way that fits who we are and the stressors we face. Even though the study of medicine fits into concrete textbooks, we as human beings don't. For real life health, it's up to each individual to have a connection with his or her body and its functioning and to consider this a priority.

The reason why symptoms tend to occur in clusters is because the different systems and processes in the body are closely connected and affect each other. In this book, we'll focus a lot on mind-body connections as well as inter-system connections in health that can often be overlooked when it comes to chronic symptoms. Let's look at a couple of examples.

The adrenal system, which deals with stress, can affect the immune system. That's why a tired and stressed body, with depleted levels of the stress hormone called cortisol, is more susceptible to colds and allergies. Stress can affect the immune system in other ways too, such as in triggering a hyperactive immune response and autoimmune illness. We'll talk more in depth about the effects stress can have on the immune system in later chapters.

Stress and emotions are also connected to the digestive system. Did you know that a part of the nervous system actually lives in the digestive tract? People sometimes feel anxiety first in their gut, showing us how thoughts and emotions are quickly communicated to the digestion. Chronic stress and suppressed emotions can derail the smooth functioning of the digestive organs, creating symptoms like heartburn, bloating, constipation, and irritable bowel.

There are countless other examples. As you will see, nothing is isolated and existing on its own island in the body. Chemical messengers in the body called hormones and neurotransmitters make sure that the different systems can communicate effectively. This is a good thing, so that the body can make adjustments in response to external and internal factors. The body's internal dialogue also makes it possible for you to adapt as an individual to changing circumstances.

It also means that we're not off the hook when we stop taking care of ourselves and ignoring our stress levels and emotions. Becoming familiar with the body's connections helps us to better support them for improved health, increased energy, and more "umph" in life. This support is important for preventive health, so that future illness can be potentially avoided, but it can also help improve any existing symptoms and conditions. Hard to treat conditions such as fibromyalgia, chronic fatigue syndrome, and Lyme disease can all benefit from this approach. In addition, common conditions such as hypertension, diabetes, thyroid dysfunction, high cholesterol, and even anxiety and depression that are typically treated with pharmaceuticals can show vast improvement from a supportive lifestyle and connection to one's own health.

So, when to start? Now. It's too easy to put it off until tomorrow, and then repeat this habit day after day. After observing my own health habits, those of my patients, and those of people I know—I've seen that when it comes to paying more attention to health, either you do it or you don't. No one is going to make you do it, not even your doctor. It has to matter to you. If you start now, you can experience the benefits of increased energy, looking and feeling better, reduced or completely resolved symptoms, and more vitality—that much sooner.

Let's get started. This book:

- Talks about the underlying mind-body connections in health,
- Describes how supporting health is an innate ability we can tap into,
- Shows how to pay better attention to the body and its signals,
- Discusses how chronic symptoms are often

related to one another,

- Describes the role of lifestyle in how we feel,
- Points out that there is no such thing as "perfect" health,
- Talks about the effects of control and suppression on the body,
- Discusses the role that fear plays in health,
- Shows how enjoyment of life is medicinal,
- Approaches autoimmunity from a new perspective,
- Demonstrates how personality ties in with how we approach our health,
- Explores why fatigue is so common today,
- Discusses how labels can be limits in getting healthy, and
- Helps bring you back to the core of your health.

Most importantly, this book can help spark curiosity and the desire to keep learning about your health so that getting healthy can be enjoyable rather than a chore. It encourages you to think about your health on a deeper level, one that resonates with you as an individual. Health is a process and you never know what you'll learn about yourself as you take better care of yourself and your body. Developing a true connection with your health helps you take full advantage of this learning process.

It takes some selfishness to find health again. "Selfish" is usually seen as a bad word, but without selfishness, it becomes difficult to make the space and time available that's needed to attend to your health. You may end up feeling like you have to be there for others more than for yourself. You may consistently put other tasks ahead of your health. Sure, there are unhealthy sides to selfishness that can involve self-absorption and hurting others. But there is also a separate and useful side of selfishness that helps us prioritize our health and be there for ourselves. Selfishness is an essential part of regaining balance in health. Being "selfish" is really just another way of saying "taking care of your *self.*"

Remember that it takes *time, patience, and practice* to regain balance in health. Doctors have practices where they see patients, but each of us as individuals have our own health practices too. They're made up of the things we do on a regular basis to take care of ourselves, both body and mind. **The more we see health as a practice rather than as a problem to fix, the more we encourage the body's natural potential to be healthy.**

Outside of the formulaic approach of the medical

system, we can each focus on more of our health than is possible during a typical health visit. We can take a look not just at how we live in terms of diet, sleep, and exercise, but also *the way we live.* The way we live involves how we choose to face unique challenges, deal with stress and disappointments, go after what we want in life, and value ourselves and our health. The typical image of "success" and "making it" in society encourages us to value many things above ourselves and our health. In your own health practice, you get a chance to look closely at these ideals and decide whether they are allowing health to thrive or blocking it. If there are things that are more important to you in life, you can re-prioritize and better support them.

The goal of this book isn't to fix digestion, sleep, stress levels, energy, and hormone balance overnight by making 50 lifestyle changes all at once. What is more effective is to learn to pay better attention to your body and to make health a real priority. If you feel inspired to make healthy lifestyle changes, try and pick one or two *accessible* ones. Accessible means that the change complements you as a person and your lifestyle. Also, think small steps. Introducing something small into your life on a consistent basis is often more effective than taking a large step only a few times. When it comes to health, the simpler the better!

We're almost ready to start painting the art of

health, but before we do I'll point out that this isn't your typical health-related book. There are no magic solutions in these chapters toward feeling and looking better. I also don't have any quick fixes or in-the-moment health fads to offer. I believe that there is medicine far more powerful and long-lasting than that, and it lies in you as a unique individual and how you choose to live. Are you going to let health be a part of your journey through life?

In making this book, I'd like to thank the patients I've seen for giving me the opportunity to continuously learn about the art of health. A huge thanks to my editor and sounding board for all things real in health, Jason Petersen, N.D. And thank you, the reader, for turning these pages and thereby being open to seeing health in a new way.

Now, let's talk about roots.

# GETTING AT YOUR UNDERLYING ROOTS

One of the principles of naturopathic medicine lies in *discovering and treating the underlying cause* of illness, rather than simply treating the isolated symptom. This is an important shift from conventional, or allopathic medicine, which focuses on treating the symptom or disease taken out of context from the rest of the body.

What this principle says in a nutshell is that you can't just put a superficial or suppressive band-aid on symptoms and expect them not to resurface. The actual cause of the illness is most important to treat for long-term health and prevention. However, is there always just one cause for an illness?

To search for one specific cause, how many lab tests and other exams need to be performed? What is the financial cost to a patient to find this exact cause, and to what extent will the information help develop a more effective treatment plan? How much time will it take for this cause to surface, and what should a patient do in the meantime?

These are all questions I've asked myself as a practicing naturopathic doctor, but also as an individual patient using both conventional and alternative health care systems. My exploration of these questions has affected the decisions I make when seeing health care providers, but even more so the decisions I make when taking care of my health at home and in daily life. The question is: What's the most helpful way to explore the root of illness while also taking action to feel better?

What I've seen from my own health and that of patients is that *the underlying triggering of symptoms is often multifaceted.* For example, one of my patients, a 38-year-old woman who we'll call Linda, experienced a period of prolonged stress and major life transition that started six months prior to her initial appointment. Around that time, Linda's business had grown very busy all of a sudden, which she was extremely happy about. On the other hand, it gave her less time to herself as she tried to juggle both family and her increasing business success.

A chain of lifestyle events started to affect Linda's overall health. While Linda enjoyed the new traffic to her business, not to mention the opportunity to hone her craft, she ended up with less time to herself than she had previously. She ate on the go, thought about her long list of things to do even during down time, and always felt in a rush. Her sugar and caffeine cravings increased in relation to stress, but Linda felt compelled to consume these things to feed her lacking energy level. Sleep, even eight hours of it, never felt like enough to replenish her energy as she was always on the go.

After a while, Linda got used to ignoring her increasing stress altogether because it had been there for so long. She grew more irritable toward others and herself. Her business was very important to her, so she didn't feel like she had the time to slow down and deal with other areas of her life. She also assumed that the stress would remain high no matter what she did.

She managed to keep up with her To-do list, but her energy was beginning to feel low all day long. After a few months, Linda developed flares of persistent and itchy eczema on her face, along with allergies. While she had a history of eczema behind her knees as a child, she had never experienced symptoms quite like these flare-ups before. She had also never dealt with seasonal allergies that wouldn't resolve with common over-the-counter medications.

What is the one specific cause of Linda's eczema? *There isn't just one.* Her symptoms are the product of real life events and the effects stress had on her lifestyle choices, energy level, immune system, overall health, and ultimately her skin. The eczema is also an outcome of how Linda chose to deal with the stress and emotions that were building up over time. Rather than just one cause, **the eczema has underlying roots that came together to trigger it.** Roots from chronic stress, roots from lifestyle choices like lack of rest and eating on the go, and roots from suppressed emotions. The roots are more accessible for treatment than the "one underlying cause," which may not even exist. Linda can address and work on her chronic stress levels, her lifestyle choices, and her suppressed emotions. Those roots are available to her on a daily basis.

Applying a cortisone cream on the skin may make Linda's symptoms go away, but the roots leading to her symptoms will still persist. As long as they do, they can sprout new symptoms in other areas of the body. The cream can eventually stop working or the suppressed skin symptoms may rebel and get worse.

Many people assume turning to a natural product or medicine is the solution, but using natural skin care alone won't take care of Linda's health roots either. The products may not work as well as they could if the roots were taken care of first. Linda may go visit a bunch of different doctors who run tests on food sensitivities and other types of labs. However, the outcome of these tests probably still won't address the actual roots. Linda may try a food elimination diet, staying away from foods that the labs show she's sensitive to. Occasionally with this type of diet, someone can have a complete resolution of symptoms, but many notice no improvement or mild to moderate improvement that doesn't last beyond a few months. Restrictive diets can also be difficult to maintain for the long-term, and they sometimes suck the joy out of eating.

How about acupuncture, massages, natural supplements, hormone treatments, a gym plan, an aesthetician who can provide facials, energy work, specialty products from dermatologists, etc? After a while, Linda might start to feel like she's just stabbing in the dark, trying treatment after treatment without rhyme or reason. This cycle is a common one people go through when dealing with chronic symptoms, and it can be frustrating.

It's not that the above treatments can't work for Linda. These modalities and medicines exist for a reason, because they can serve as a bridge toward better health. They just have less chance of working in a healthy and long-standing way if Linda doesn't slow down and attend to her health roots as well. As long as Linda neglects the roots that sprouted her eczema in the first place, her symptoms run the risk of resurfacing or getting worse, no matter what treatments she tries out.

> # Challenge Question:
>
> *Which roots might be the source of your health symptoms?*
>
> *To help you think about this question in-depth, try drawing out what you see on a piece of paper in the form of a tree. The roots are the underlying causes while the branches are the chronic symptoms you are having.*

**The best health outcomes happen when the individual comes before the treatment, and not the other way around.** Each person's health is unique, and so is the story (a.k.a. the roots) of their symptoms. If you place all the emphasis on a single underlying cause or the exact treatment you're using for a symptom, you can easily forget what types of roots created the symptom in the first place.

The roots are uniquely tied to who you are, your personality, your situation, and your experience. Even if the symptom itself starts to get better from treatment, if the roots are neglected you risk having the symptom return or turn up in a different form. Even more important than the symptom returning, you miss the opportunity to learn about and attend to your overall health.

As mentioned in the Challenge Question, if the underlying causes are the roots of illness, then the symptoms could be seen as the branches that you see above the surface. Healthy roots lead to healthy branches. Each symptom the body sends us is like a unique signal letting us know that the body needs more support. The symptom lets us know that one or more health imbalances are happening and it's time to pay attention to them. They're the clues that can help lead you toward better health, if you follow their trail. In the next section, we'll talk about just that—how to pay better attention to your body and the signals it's trying to send you.

# PAYING ATTENTION TO THE BODY'S "SIGNALS"

What do we tend to want most when a symptom pops up in the body? We want it to disappear, pronto. There's often a feeling that we "just don't want to deal with it." A thought may even pop up that sounds like "I don't have time for this." If this sounds familiar to you, you're not alone. There is often a lot going on in each person's life, and it makes sense that health symptoms aren't a welcome guest.

On the other hand, this is the body we're talking about, and it tries to communicate imbalances in health by using symptoms. The body—that gets us up each morning so we can make money, go get an education, or make breakfast for our families. The one that makes walking, running, breathing, and eating possible. It spikes those volleyballs for us, lands the 8-ball in the game winning pocket, bears children, gets us grooving to a fun beat.

It's also the one that tries to process our thoughts, emotions, and stress so that they don't build up and wreak havoc on the nervous system and other organs. The body handles daily wear and tear, eight hours of work, standing or sitting for long periods of time. It makes socializing possible, and reading, and thinking. Is the body something we really want to shut out of our lives and not have enough time for? If that's a decision we make, what will the body say in return? It probably won't be too happy about that choice.

Like we touched on before, **symptoms are the body's way of communicating information about what's going on with its functions.** Let's think about how cars work for a moment. Cars have sensors that read how a vehicle is running and they'll let you know if the engine is over-heating, whether the gas needs refilled, if your seatbelt is unbuckled, when the oil pressure is too low, if it's time to check the engine, as well as tons of other important information. We need the sensors' signals because they let us know about the internal functioning of the car. We don't have x-ray vision to see what's going on under the hood while the car's running, so sensors pick up info about what's not working and relay it to us.

The body also has sensors that relay information about stress levels, nutrition, organ function, and other physiological processes. For example, two of the body's sensors include heart rate and blood pressure, which your doctor checks. There are a variety of other "sensors" that you can keep track of at home too, and these sensors offer *detectable* information about how the body's doing. They also let us know whether the body needs more support for its health. Sometimes when life gets busy, we can get used to chronic symptoms and stress as being "normal" without even realizing it. For example, have you ever suddenly noticed that your shoulders are tense and they're hiked up almost to your ears?

It helps to check in with the body's sensors from time to time so that chronic symptoms and stress don't become the norm. Without taking a break and doing this, the speed of daily living can take over and prioritize everything else over how we're feeling. **Next you'll find some of the sensors you can check in with, along with common signals—or symptoms (sx)—in each area.** Keep in mind that this is not an exhaustive list and you may think of other sensors and signals as you read through these examples.

# The Body's Sensors and Signals

**1) Energy level**
- sx: Fatigue, low energy, sugar and/or caffeine cravings, irritability, weak immune system, low libido

**2) Sleep patterns**
- sx: Trouble falling asleep, difficulty staying asleep, erratic sleep schedule, mood swings

**3) Mental clarity**
- sx: Difficulty concentrating, attention deficit, foggy mind, memory issues

**4) Appetite levels**
- sx: Low appetite, emotional eating, overeating, sugar and carbohydrate cravings

**5) Digestion**
- sx: Heartburn, nausea, upset stomach, gas, bloating, moodiness

**6) Elimination**
- sx: Constipation, diarrhea, acne or other skin issues, lowered or hypersensitive immune system

## 7) Breathing

- sx:  Shortness of breath, low stamina, tight chest muscles, anxiety

## 8) Immunity

- sx:  Frequent colds, flu, chronic allergies, skin conditions like eczema, autoimmunity

## 9) Mood

- sx: Anxiety, depression, irritability, nervousness, big ups and downs

## 10) Motivation

- sx: Low drive, loss of interest in activities, apathy, low libido

## 11) Cravings

- sx: Reliance on sugar, caffeine, nicotine, or another substance for its effects on body

## 12) Weight

- sx: Overweight or underweight, midsection (belly) weight gain, sluggishness, joint pain

## 13) Skin

- sx: Acne, eczema, rosacea, psoriasis, sensitive skin, overly dry or oily skin, inflammation

## 14) Hair and nails

- sx: Dry, brittle, weakness or breaking, unexplained hair loss, pitted or lined nails

## 15) Muscular tension in the body

- sx: Tight neck and shoulders, low back pain, clenched jaw, headaches or migraines

## 16) Menstrual cycles (for women)

- sx: PMS, cramps, moodiness, irritability, sugar cravings, bloating

## 17) Hormone levels

- sx: Fatigue, hot flashes, night sweats, weight gain, mood swings, low libido, cold hands and feet, rapid aging

## 18) Libido

- sx: Low sex drive, low energy, low motivation, difficulty getting or maintaining erection

## 19) Inflammation

- sx: Musculoskeletal pain, joint soreness, red and inflamed skin conditions, weight gain

## 20) Cardiovascular system

- sx: Rapid heart rate, irregular heartbeat, heart pain, cold hands and feet, headaches

## 21) Mental

- sx: Racing thoughts, worries and doubts that get worse the more you think about them, "stuck" ways of thinking

---

# Exercise:

As you run down this list, write down which sensors have been sending you signals to pay attention to.

---

Each of these sensors sends us information every day in an easy-to-read way. Let's look at a snapshot of what balanced health would look like in each area, sensor by sensor. When things are running fairly smoothly:

- We have energy to do the things we want to do
- We fall asleep fairly easily and enjoy a full night's rest

- We feel relatively refreshed in the morning and motivated to start the day
- The mind is able to concentrate when it needs to
- Memory is available when needed
- A healthy appetite brings on predictable hunger signals, alerting us of meal times
- Food is digested and waste is eliminated smoothly, without chronic gas, bloating, or constipation
- Belly breathing happens naturally, and breath doesn't become trapped by tense chest muscles
- The immune system can mostly defend against and resolve allergies and colds
- The mood experiences natural shifts, depending on how the day goes, but each feeling doesn't become paralyzing
- Stress is mostly managed and any cravings for sugar, caffeine, and nicotine don't get out of control
- Belly weight is regulated, so that pants buttons can relax and not worry about popping off
- Skin, hair, and nails are strong and hydrated
- Skin boundary feels strong and healthy without chronic eruptions, sensitivity, irritation, and redness (inflammation)
- Muscular tension is manageable and not too

knotty, especially in the neck, shoulders, and upper back

- Menstrual cycles (for women) are fairly regular in timing and with only mild PMS, if any
- Hormones are in balance and symptoms like hot flashes, night sweats, mood swings, low libido, and weight gain are improved or absent
- Libido feels healthy, enjoyable, and satisfying
- Inflammation is low in the body, and joints can move freely without chronic and unrelenting pain
- No chronic headaches from tension or stress
- Heart rhythm is regular and steady
- Hands and feet are warm

If you recognized one or more sensors that have been alerting you to pay more attention to health, the next thought may surface as, "Okay—what do I do next to solve it?" Hold off on that thought. Health isn't just about fixing what's wrong, and the fixing mentality can often lead us to search for magic treatments rather than to look at our own unique and underlying roots of health.

Behind the sensor that's beeping, there is often a chain of events that led up to that particular symptom. If there are a few different sensors going off at once, there is probably an underlying pattern to which organ systems are communicating the information. Finding the pattern helps you know where to start with healthier approaches to lifestyle, rather than simply seeking to put a band-aid on the sensor and "fixing it" with a temporary treatment. Most of us, after slowing down to pay attention to our health, would choose a long-term approach to improving a symptom rather than a quick, but merely short-term solution.

Let's look at an example of sensors in action. A 45-year-old woman named Susan scheduled an appointment to see me about her weight gain of six months, particularly around the belly area. No matter how much Susan exercised, which included at least an hour at the gym five days a week, the belly weight was not shedding a pound. Susan had also worked on improving her diet, which was already mostly healthy with daily home-cooked meals. Her dietary changes included consuming less fat and cutting out refined sugar and carbohydrates wherever possible. Still, no change in belly weight. Susan was getting frustrated with her lack of success. She enjoyed the health benefits of exercising and eating well, but she also wanted to look good and prevent future illness that can be associated with increased abdominal fat.

While talking with Susan about her weight, we uncovered other sensors that were sending signals to her as well. Susan's energy felt low, except immediately after workouts. She was also experiencing insomnia with racing thoughts. Tearfulness and depression were getting worse around her menstrual cycle, along with increased bloating and mood swings. Even outside of her menstrual cycle, Susan felt irritable toward her family and her moods were unpredictable, which she wasn't historically used to. Something was clearly blocking Susan's weight loss efforts as well as her overall health.

---

### Susan's Signals

Midsection Weight Gain
Insomnia
Tearfulness
Mood Swings
Bloating
Low Energy
Racing Thoughts at Night
Depression
PMS
Irritability

---

As we talked about the onset (starting point) of Susan's cluster of symptoms, she started to reveal what was going on in her life at the time. She had just moved to the Bay Area and was transitioning to new work and social environments. Susan and her family had previously lived in a smaller and more slow-paced town and after the move, life started feeling more rushed. She didn't spend much time to herself outside of her daily workout session in the morning.

Most of her time was spent caring for her family during the changes. Overall, Susan's stress was building while constantly worrying about others and neglecting herself in the process. Life circumstances and Susan's mentality made it hard for her to pay attention to her body's signals.

Susan didn't have to think much about these factors before identifying them out loud. She was intuitively aware of what was going on in her life to disrupt her health, but life had felt so busy since her family's relocation that she put her stress, symptoms, and needed self care on the backburner in order to be a rock for her family. Susan's family was also starting to notice the changes in her health.

While Susan had taken steps to do all the "right things" to be healthy, such as eating well and exercising, she still had a nagging feeling that her health was out of balance overall. She was right. All of us have an innate understanding of what prevents us from taking care of ourselves, but we often choose to ignore it, especially when life gets busy and stressful...which can feel like pretty much every day for many people!

Even though Susan's treatment plan involved natural therapies, supplements, and lifestyle modifications aimed at balancing hormone levels and increasing energy, they were not the cornerstone of her treatment. For Susan, front and center was the recommendation that she allot more time to herself as a person who deserves to be healthy and to be taken care of just as much as she was used to taking care of others.

In the office, we discussed the importance of slowing down and paying attention to her body's sensors and the signals they were sending her. **Using these signals, she could tell when it was time for her to take better care of herself.** We also talked about how unacknowledged stress was affecting each area of her health.

Her daily exercise was a good start for de-stressing both the body and mind, but we also focused on "in the moment" relaxation techniques such as deep breathing, stretching, and a simple exercise where Susan could stop and ask herself "How do I feel right now?" Months of worrying and stressing had taxed Susan's adrenal glands, which lab testing of cortisol levels further proved was the case. We had her start an adrenal support formula to strengthen her adrenal glands and balance energy levels.

We also needed to address Susan's sleep disturbance signal, as restful sleep supports healthy weight. She tried some muscular and breathing relaxation techniques to deepen her quality of sleep, along with starting a natural sleep aid that could serve as a bridge toward better sleep. Quality rest, uninterrupted by racing thoughts and worries, would let Susan's body replenish hormones that are needed for weight regulation.

At first, Susan felt she didn't have the time to approach her health in this comprehensive way, but with practice she became more comfortable and used to paying attention to the symptoms she was having. As she listened more carefully to her body's signals, she was able to relax more and her symptoms naturally started to improve. At Susan's follow-up visits, she reported not only feeling better in terms of her body's signals (a.k.a. her symptoms), but also seeing a big difference in her midsection weight. Improved energy, restful sleep, balanced hormones, and attention to stress levels were all supporting healthier weight. Though Susan previously held doubts, she actively worked on putting herself first and trusting that her family would be okay while she shifted priorities a bit. To her surprise, it turned out that her family welcomed these changes too!

---

# Challenge Question:

*After reading about Susan's journey with her health, what do you think is the most important change she made?*

---

Often we think of specific treatments as the main solution to health complaints. In Susan's case, she made a different and farther-reaching discovery by acknowledging that *she and her health should come first.* She learned that by paying attention to her body's sensors and their respective signals, she could actually communicate back to her body and improve how she felt by taking better care of herself.

She also saw the "big picture" of her health, in that each signal that her body was sending was not isolated or random. The symptoms that she was experiencing as a cluster were related, and therefore her efforts toward self care helped improve multiple symptoms (or signals) at once. Finally, Susan understood that the potential for health was a natural ability that she could harness.

Think about how much space you allow in your life to pay attention to the signals that your body sends you. We often neglect our body's signals in favor of a go-go mentality. However, these signals are the essential clues that we can follow, much like a detective, toward better health! In many ways, they tell us more than lab results can at the doctor's office. By paying attention to these clues, we acknowledge the body's health as a top priority. In the long run, this mentality helps us live life without burning out and taxing the health of the body.

---

# Exercise:

Find a pencil and a piece of paper. Close your eyes for a moment and with each exhale, loosen any tension in your neck, shoulders, chest, arms, forearms, and hands. Once you feel grounded in your body, go from head-to-toe and make a note of which areas (or sensors) are asking you to pay more attention to them. Even if the sensor isn't sending a signal this exact moment, try and recall if in the past month it's been communicating with you on a frequent basis. Remember, not all signals are strictly physical in nature. Some are mood- and energy-related, so be open to any fatigue, anxiety, nervousness, irritability, or depression. When you're ready, slowly open your eyes and write down the signals you paid attention to.

The very act of paying attention to your body's signals is what allows the healing process to begin. Ignoring the signals is what blocks the potential for health, which can lead to a domino effect of neglected health. If we each have an innate ability to communicate with our health in this manner, why don't we just do it? As we learned from Susan's example, it's often the stress, pressures, expectations, ideals, and sometimes "problems" (that aren't always real problems) in life that lead us to ignore what is already apparent to us. With practice, you can become more familiar with your body's signals so that if they arise, you will know that it's time to take action and take better care of yourself.

In Susan's case, we explored how ignoring the body's signals during stress can noticeably disrupt health, especially when there is a lack of down time to rest in between. We can't eliminate all stress from life because stress is a part of reality for everyone. But we can make some adjustments to decrease the impact that stress has on overall health and the sensors we just covered. Let's look at the ins and outs of stress in the next section, along with the art of relaxation.

# THE THREE R'S AND ONE P OF HEALTH

We've all had a cold before. The sneezing, coughing, sore throat, runny nose, and run down feeling is familiar to each person and so is the common recommendation to get rest during a cold. No matter what health care system you visit, the suggestion to rest during a cold is a standard. Rest is the activity that feels most comfortable when we're sick, so this advice feels welcome and natural to us. In fact, a part of us may even enjoy the opportunity to rest despite the cold, and we may even feel a twinge of sadness once the cold resolves completely and life picks up at its usual and relentlessly fast pace again. The question becomes, if rest feels so good for the body during a cold, why don't we employ it for health on a regular basis or when we're experiencing other symptoms?

**We may not be taking rest seriously enough as a solid approach to health and prevention.** A common contributor to chronic health conditions in this day and age is *stress.* Stress may sound like a vague concept, but its effects are real and substantial. We all know of its presence in life and how it makes us feel when it gets out of control. In fact, lab values of the stress hormone, cortisol, frequently show up out of balance in my patients who report high stress.

Patients also commonly describe worsening of symptoms such as flare ups of acne, increased insomnia, more digestive issues, uncontrollable allergies, intense sugar cravings, and heightened mood swings during times of high stress. Rather than being an impartial spectator in the body, stress is an active participant in how it affects hormones, neurotransmitters, and the functioning of the body's organ systems. Just because everyone has stress doesn't mean that it makes sense to ignore this important factor in quality of health and daily living.

We can't make stress disappear, but we don't need to in order to find balance in health. The three R's of personal health care and the one P include: *Rest, Relaxation, Rejuvenation, and Pampering.* If all of these words sound foreign to your present lifestyle, that's okay. You have to start somewhere. Many of us don't take time out for these important healthful activities, which are all related. The reasons we explain to ourselves for not taking them seriously may sound like excuses after we actually try them. Just like health can be easy to put at the back of the line in life, the role of the three R's and P often gets put back there as well. You may be surprised to hear that being busy is not the only reason we tend to do this. **It's also because relaxing can be scary and challenging at first.**

What's so scary about resting and relaxing? A few things. Not all of our occupied time is spent doing work, and some or most of it easily gets filled with distractions. Distractions can be anything from checking social media ten times a day to worrying incessantly about a small issue. Distractions are okay in moderation, but in excess they can become a method to avoid dealing with what we're going through and how we're feeling.

Rest and relaxation can feel daunting at first because they put us face to face with not only our health and bodies, but also with those things we've been trying to avoid in life using time-filling distractions. In addition to feeling good and supporting our bodies, relaxation brings us a more honest perspective on ourselves and life. This perspective can feel like a mental shift as it brings more clearly to the forefront the real challenges we're going through.

## Challenge Questions:

*1) What types of distractions have been filling up a lot of your time?*

*2) Taking a step back, how important are these distractions to you for your overall life?*

*3) How could these distractions be affecting your health?*

Another common reason that we fear resting, relaxing, rejuvenating, and pampering is the message, either internally or externally delivered, that it's forbidden to put ourselves first in this way. We may subconsciously be convinced that we don't deserve this luxury and must instead run ourselves ragged going, going, going in a quest to prove ourselves in one way or another. We may place a lot of unreasonable pressure and expectations on ourselves that are impossible to meet. Therefore, the proper time to rest and relax can never arrive until these expectations are met (which they never will be). It can be scary to bring expectations down to a more doable level, be less hard on ourselves, and enjoy the relaxation that we do deserve in both health and life.

One other factor that deters us from relaxing is the tendency to compare ourselves and our lives to those around us. We may focus on how busy and accomplished everyone else seems, concluding that rest is not a wise decision if we want to keep up with everyone else. Do we really know what everyone else is doing? No, but the human mind has a habit of making comparisons and harboring the fear of lagging behind everyone else.

If this habit of comparison plays like a broken record in your life, take a moment and let yourself fully admit that you're thinking this way. Often, we can get so used to comparing ourselves to others that we're not even aware we're doing it. It's not necessary to fix the issue in your mind, but rather to *slowly figure out what you really want to do despite what anyone else is doing.* The act itself of going for what you want leaves less space for comparisons, and even when they do come up it will get easier to see them for what they are and to move forward anyway.

To allow more rest and relaxation into your life, you have to get used to putting yourself first more than you might be used to. Putting yourself first means that your time is yours, your actions are yours, and your decisions are yours. In other words, you allow yourself the freedom to give your body and mind what they need in that moment no matter what else is going on.

Why? **Because you want to.** So often, we go without the things we want in life because of guilt that arises surrounding doing things our own way. We may fear that those around us won't approve of the changes we make, because they're used to us acting in a particular way. We may feel we're neglecting important responsibilities or others who need us. When these types of feelings come up, it's natural. Changes, even good ones like taking more time to relax in life, set in gradually and they take courage too. Just because fears come up doesn't mean it's time to give up or that you're silly for having these emotions. This is part of the learning process for anyone wanting to feel healthier.

You don't have to be on a beach or at a luxury spa to relax. Relaxing can be very simple and tailored to fit whatever amount of time you have available for it. Everyone is different, so what you choose for relaxing will be unique to you. You may decide to take a short nap, read a book while drinking chamomile tea, do a session of yoga or tai chi, go for a walk, play music, or write. If you notice muscle tightness in your neck and shoulders, you can take a relaxing bath. If you only have ten minutes, you can do some deep belly breathing to calm the nervous system. You can enjoy a piece of dark chocolate. Listen to some music. Get a little sun. Do some simple stretching. Be as creative as you want, it's your time!

Carving "me time" into life is valuable, as we saw in the last section with Susan's case. It's nice to be around other people, but without any alone time it can become challenging to get real relaxation and practice better health. This personal time allows us to release stress, get in touch with how we're feeling, and often to get perspective on life. As stress lowers and becomes more manageable, we encourage our adrenal and nervous systems to calm down and strike more balance. The body can then naturally experience improvement of chronic symptoms such as fatigue, digestive issues, skin complaints, trouble sleeping, mood swings, and low libido. The body has an innate healing ability that gets a boost from the three R's and P.

Outside of rest and relaxation, Me Time can involve other creative elements too including rejuvenation and pampering. Trying something new in life can feel rejuvenating, such as learning a new hobby or visiting a new place. Stepping out of your comfort zone once in a while opens up both the body and mind to learning, and it can spark vitality in health as well. When we get stuck in familiarity of the same routine day after day, energy can get stuck too whether we're aware of it or not. Introducing some fresh and new experiences can shake things up just enough so that you're open to life in a new way, and often a needed way.

Pampering also has therapeutic potential, even though on the outside it might seem frivolous at first. Do you ever notice the feeling you have after getting a new haircut? You feel different, and lighter. Maybe you get a stimulating scalp massage during the wash that feels relaxing. After your hairdresser is finished and hands you a mirror, you notice that you not only look different, but you also look healthier! Pampering allows you to both feel and look good, promoting overall health. Check out more pampering tips in the next Exercise box, and you can also brainstorm some on your own.

# Exercise:

Here are simple steps you can take at home to pamper yourself:

1. Massage soothing lotion or oil into your calves and feet to increase circulation and muscle relaxation.
2. Gently brush your arms and legs with a dry skin brush (from tips toward the heart) to exfoliate and get lymph flowing. Take a shower and drink water afterward.
3. Take care of your nails, hands, and feet by giving yourself a simple manicure or pedicure.
4. Try a facial mask and apply cucumber slices to the eyes.
5. Clean out your closet and switch up your style for a refreshing change.

*Whatever you try, you'll see the benefits to your health almost immediately!*

In my own health, I've seen that when stress and pressures start building up, that's the time during which it's easiest to ignore the three R's and P.

Interestingly, that's also the time when these simple techniques can be most effective in helping alleviate stress and pressure. Ironic, huh? Sometimes we tend to ignore the very medicine we need, even when it's staring us straight in the face. The simplest approaches in health can often prove to be the most powerful. When your mind is trying to tell you that you're too stressed to deal with your stress, that's the best time to turn to the three R's and P for a little help.

In this section, we touched on how fear can play a part in health. Fear is a real factor that arises both when we feel imbalances in our health and as we're trying to get healthier. It can affect the decisions we make about health, increase stress about our symptoms, and paralyze our efforts toward feeling better. In the next section, we'll elaborate more on this topic and talk about how to prevent fear from getting the best of your health.

# THE PART FEAR PLAYS IN HEALTH

A big factor that can cripple an individual's power to find health is—FEAR. We've all seen the faces of fear in the arena of health, and by now we may be so used to their messages that we seldom pause to question them. Research may come out about the terrible things that can happen down the road if you eat eggs or drink coffee. All of a sudden, you feel fear ripple through your blood as you take inventory of how long and how frequently you've been eating those Egg McMuffins or drinking your Venti Starbucks coffees. The research emphasizes all the health problems that can come about, so you vow never to consume those evildoers again. You don't notice a change in your health over time, but hey, at least you're being safe.

Even though this scenario is just one example of how fear can affect our health-related actions and decisions, health care tends to be riddled with many triggers of fear that can take residence in our own minds. Instead of inspiring us and motivating us toward health, fear can exert the opposite effect. It often stops us in our tracks, leading us to question every move we make in health and even in life.

Fearful and neurotic thoughts can introduce a bunch of unnecessary rules into our lives, including many neon "Forbidden" signs in our minds. These thoughts may sound like:

- Wait, that commercial says that my blood pressure is uncontrollable without this new medication? I better ask my doctor to prescribe it!
- Oh no, my friend said that chocolate causes acne. No more chocolate for me, sigh.
- I tried a latte with dairy the other day, and my eczema flared. I can't drink that ever again, because it causes my skin symptoms.
- My doctor doesn't sound optimistic about my condition, so what's the use in trying to get better?
- Diabetes runs in my family, and since it can be genetic, I'm probably going to get it too no matter what I do.
- I heard that gluten and dairy are bad and everyone's staying away from it. I should also cut it out.
- The air outside is toxic? Oh no, I breathed

that air, so what will happen to me now?
- My lab results weren't completely normal, my health must be in bad shape.

---

## **Challenge Questions:**

*Are there fears that have been dominating your thoughts regarding your health? If so, what are they?*

---

The list of health-related fears goes on indefinitely. It's natural to experience some worries or fears when symptoms come up or when we don't feel our best. What we want to avoid is allowing this fear to control how we live and our overall beliefs about getting better. **Remember, the body has an inborn ability to support health and heal itself, and many chronic symptoms come about when we neglect our bodies and our lifestyles. Fear is often a strong influence in creating or perpetuating this neglect.**

Much of the potential to feel better lies in you as a person and the choices you make about your health. When we get overly fearsome, worrisome, and superstitious about health, these feelings can override our ability to pay better attention to our bodies. In a big way, these fear-based habits can stop, limit, or even reverse our efforts to become healthier. They also contribute to increased stress, which can further upset the body's overall balance in health. In this way, ironically, even "positive" actions towards health, when motivated by fear, can actually be detrimental to health.

Where do fears about health come from? They can come from anywhere and we're almost raised from a young age to fear all things related to health. The word "health" in fact can start to immediately trigger thoughts about "disease" or "illness" in people's minds rather than a desire to pay attention to how we're feeling and to connect with the body. That might be why the last time many people remember learning about health or the body is during sixth grade health class. Unfortunately, the fear surrounding health can give this important topic a hands-off reputation that it doesn't deserve.

The encouraged overreliance on the medical system to tell us what healthy means doesn't help the situation either. For certain facets of the medical community, pharmaceutical industry, and insurance system, fear surrounding health is taken advantage of for marketing purposes and to establish greater authority. In these cases, the emphasis is usually not on people learning about and understanding their health.

It's about people knowing less and fearing more, so the system can run smoothly and people are more swayed to buy what's being advertised and peddled without questions. We have to remain cognizant when fear-based messages about health are thrown our way, whether from the medical community, people we know, drug commercials, the news at night, or our own minds.

The type of mindset we have toward health affects how we feel. On the one hand, it can help us feel motivated to be healthy and live life the way we want. On the opposite end, it can scare us, make us feel worse, and discourage us from practicing the art of health or living our lives. Let's look at an example of how fear can affect health on a real level.

A 57-year-old man named Mike scheduled an appointment to see me for his hypertension. He was concerned not only about his condition, but also about the blood pressure medication he was taking and the manner in which it was prescribed five months prior. Mike felt perturbed that his doctor didn't ask questions about his lifestyle before prescribing a drug, but he went ahead and started taking the medication as directed. Not only did the treatment not regulate his blood pressure (which he took daily readings of), but he also started to experience what seemed like side effects.

He felt dizzy and "out of it," and he was also having unexplained numbness and tingling in his body. The blood pressure medication was supposed to have made him feel better, but he had felt worse. He started to wonder if he should try stress relief measures and other alternative approaches to health alongside his medication. He also wondered if his doctor could switch the medication to a new one that might have fewer side effects for him.

Mike had a difficult time reaching his doctor to ask about the side effects of his medication. He went ahead and scheduled a follow up appointment instead of waiting for a call back. Mike described how at the visit, the physician seemed annoyed with him for asking about stress relief and integrative health approaches for improving hypertension. The doctor also didn't have patience to go over Mike's adverse reaction to taking the drug or discuss switching prescriptions. He instead went ahead to prescribe a second blood pressure medication for Mike to try in combination with the first one.

When Mike expressed concern about having even more side effects, the doctor replied irritably that without proper treatment, Mike could end up in the emergency room or worse. He then abruptly ended the appointment after ten minutes. After his appointment, Mike felt scared, panicky, and stressed.

When Mike came to see me, he was still very stressed and afraid for his health. He really wanted to feel healthy again, but he couldn't come to terms with the possibility he'd be taking more and more medication as he got older, with potentially more unwanted side effects. The message that his health was doomed had settled in and Mike didn't know what to do next. He also didn't fill his second blood pressure prescription, not knowing how much worse he'd feel from taking two medications he knew nothing about.

We kept Mike on his first medication while also starting him on an adrenal tonic to help him manage his stress better. We also talked about stress and Mike's tendency to keep his feelings so internalized that he seldom recognized when he was getting upset or anxious. Mike realized at some point during the visit that he does get a sinking feeling in the pit of his stomach, along with a cramping pain, before or during situations that he's dreading.

The more he talked, Mike realized that it was normal to talk about health in this way and his demeanor calmed down and became less fearful. He received tailored lifestyle recommendations and natural therapies aimed at helping him manage his stress, find more balance in his hormone levels and overall health, and support healthier blood pressure. We talked about how blood pressure is just one measure of health, and rather than fixate on that alone, Mike could also gauge his health in other ways by paying more attention to his body and what he's going through.

---

## **Exercise:**

For each fear that is playing a strong role in your health, jot down a healthy step you can take that is not rooted in fear or superstition. As you write these steps down, try and envision them happening in your life.

---

At his follow-up visits, Mike's blood pressure readings improved and the panic and fear surrounding his health decreased dramatically at the same time. Mike spoke more confidently about the steps *he wanted to take* for his health and in his life. He no longer saw the medical system as owning his health and knew instead that he was in charge of how he felt and where his health was headed. At each visit, it was apparent that Mike was learning more about himself and his health and would keep doing so. He never did fill that second prescription from his previous doctor.

Mike not only became healthier and gained a better understanding of his body, but he also became more aware of fear-based messages about health. He worked on his own attitude toward health, so that it was less fear driven and more motivated by preventive measures and how he wanted to feel.

The mind is a powerful tool. It can help us in our efforts toward health or it can block our attempts using fear, superstition, and worries. How we decide to use this tool is up to each of us. Mike, for one, decided that he wasn't going to let fears get the best of his potential for health.

In the next section, let's look more closely at the mind's important role in health.

# THE POWER OF THE MIND

Try and pinpoint one area of life that is unaffected by how we think. The truth is, there isn't one! The human mind is interwoven with our day-to-day experiences and that includes our health. Without the mind, there is no daily life or health to speak of in the first place. The question is: How does this basic fact become so easily lost when we're talking about health care? Can we really feel better without paying attention to how we think?

**The mind is a powerful tool that can help us grow, learn about ourselves, and feel increased health. At the same time, it can also create obstacles on the road to better health, which happens to all of us at some point.** Because mainstream medicine focuses more attention on evidence-based research, health-related fads, cultural trends, and quick fixes, the influence of the mind on health seldom comes up in a meaningful way. When it is brought up, much of the time the emphasis is on how to suppress our thoughts, criticize ourselves for having "negative" ones, and how to keep everything in check overall:

"Take this new drug to feel less depressed or anxious."

"Think positively at all costs."

"Just be happy."

Today, random tidbits like "broccoli is packed with antioxidants" or "just think positive" can easily turn into health mantras, while a simple and common sense statement like "your mindset affects your health" is often ignored or becomes an afterthought. Why? Because it isn't promising an answer or solution. It's asking you to take a look at yourself for real clues on how you're feeling.

Broccoli may be packed with nutrients and positive thoughts may sound nice, but no amount of broccoli and positive thinking can substitute for a direct look at what you're experiencing. If we don't ask ourselves how thought patterns are affecting how we feel, we miss out on the health potential that can be unlocked from an honest look at mindset.

The power of the mind comes into play in sports, so let's use it to create a handy metaphor for health. Imagine you're an athlete, say a tennis player for example. You practice diligently, hire a great coach, perfect each tennis shot, and get in awesome shape. You're playing matches and winning. All the hard work is paying off!

Then one day, a match comes along that throws you for a loop. You're playing your best tennis ever, but nothing goes how you expected against your new opponent. On top of that, weather conditions are gusty, which you aren't prepared for. As you're nearing the end of your match (about to lose), you start to wonder whether all your hard work is for nothing and if life is against you. You ask: "What's the use?"

The match ends, you go home, and life and tennis go on. You tell yourself that "negative" thoughts about tennis are bad and are best to ignore when they come up. Instead, you'll think more "positively." After this major loss, you decide to hit the gym and the court even harder. You put even more effort than you did before into preparing a pique tennis game. You think positive thoughts no matter what and you criticize yourself when any other mindset tries to enter the picture. You're ready to get back in the game!

You easily lose your next three matches.

*What happened?*

Rather than searching for a single answer to this question, the key is to look at the situation and see that something did change. It wasn't a lack of preparation. It wasn't that you faced new opponents. It wasn't unpredictable weather conditions. And it wasn't even losing in and of itself. A challenge came up, that's for sure. A major loss is never easy to face in sports or life in general. It's how you handled the challenge that set a path for what would come next. Did the act of ignoring "negative" thoughts in favor of being chronically positive offer you a healthy approach to dealing with a loss and moving on from it?

After the next three losses, you're tired and don't feel like spending even more hours at the court and at the gym. You and your coach talk about your tennis mindset, which you discover extends beyond tennis into life itself. You've gotten used to driving yourself hard in life without any breaks, and the mentality is starting to stifle the creativity and fun of your game. You used to enjoy tennis!

You start to see that winning has become everything, and you hardly even give yourself credit for the wins anymore. Tennis now feels like an order rather than a choice, and the first loss you experienced really brought home that feeling. What seemed like bad or negative thoughts at the time were really a sign to take a step back from the wins and losses to look at the big picture of what was going on underneath. Try putting yourself in this hypothetical tennis scenario and imagining how you would like things to change before answering the following questions:

## Challenge Questions:

*1) In this tennis metaphor, how do you picture the next few matches will feel regardless of the outcome of the match?*

*2) How will the new mindset influence your overall health, both on and off the tennis court?*

It's more helpful to let thoughts naturally exist than to quickly label and categorize them as they arise. It's not easy to do this, but difficult or so-called negative thoughts aren't going to stick around forever just because you look at them. In fact, the more you allow yourself to acknowledge those thoughts, the better able you are to learn from them and the less you're inclined to let them control you. Positive thoughts, as good as they may feel in the moment, also can't stick around permanently regardless of whether they're natural or self-imposed. The mind has a more fluid nature than we usually give it credit for and thoughts aren't strictly good or bad, black or white.

Have you ever watched an after-match press conference for one of the tennis greats, such as Roger

Federer or Rafael Nadal? Whether they've just encountered a win or a loss, you can tell there are important thoughts and emotions at play during the interview that can eventually help them get where they want to go next in their careers and their lives. First, however, they have to look at what they're going through. Even with their incredible skill, neither of these players got to where they are by ignoring negative or uncomfortable thoughts in favor of 100% positivity. They harnessed the power of the mind in its many different shades of color during the challenges of loss as well as triumph, and all the times in between that other people don't see.

The tennis metaphor shows us how we can use the power of the mind toward our health. *There is a tendency in all of us to be hardest on ourselves during difficult times, when we could really benefit from being there for ourselves.* We may instead come to expect ourselves to use our thoughts to just "snap out of it" and pretend that everything is fine and unchanged. We just have to do more and be more, we tell ourselves. Or we decide we'll never be good enough anyway.

These two statements are actually opposite sides of the same coin and they effectively lock our other thoughts away in a vault. These expectations place more pressure on our lives and block the opportunity for growth, learning, and health to unfold naturally.

The beauty of the mind is that we can think for ourselves. Our thoughts don't need to be manipulated and prettied in order to be useful to us. They do need to be looked at and lived through in a real, individual, and honest way. You may be surprised to see what keys you uncover for your health when you explore your thoughts with less judgment and more curiosity.

What else does the mind have a tendency to do that can prove detrimental for health? *Control.* Rather than face the uncertainties that naturally come about in life, we often want to decide how things will turn out beforehand. Uncertainty can be scary, so we suppress our emotions surrounding it and try and control situations using mental force. What happens? We're not able to control everything and in the process of dedicating ourselves to this goal, health often suffers. In the next section, we'll talk more about the very real effect control and suppression can have on health and our bodies.

# THE ILLUSION OF CONTROL & YOUR HEALTH

As human beings, we like to try and control outcomes. That's just the way we are. When life gets stressful or change is imminent, we figure we can control ourselves and our environments to influence how things turn out and to make everything feel "fine" and "normal." The illusion of control comes at a price, however. In order to keep acting like everything's under control and figured out, we have to ignore what's really going on. We often suppress our emotions to keep the illusion going and neglect our health in the process. Controlling can become a bad habit that affects health just like any other bad habit.

Of course, there are different types of control and not all of them are inherently unhealthy. For example, when you bring much needed and healthy change to a work environment or a relationship, it can feel good to be more in control of the situation. This type of control fosters growth and learning for ourselves and those we interact with. On the flip side, control can also stem from our fears and act in a much more suppressive way. When we try to exercise tight control over outcomes, situations, and people out of fear, this behavior can not only be counterproductive, but it can also disrupt our health. This latter type of control is what we'll focus on in this section.

**Have you ever tried to exert control over yourself or your environment, only to find that you feel even more stress or anxiety afterward?** Control and suppression don't feel natural and we have to put a great deal of effort into maintaining them. They also don't make stress go away, only creating a temporary illusion of no stress. Underneath the image we create, we still feel the anxieties, worries, and fears trying to break through to the surface. The mind is very powerful in its ability to suppress, so the neglected emotions keep bubbling underground and can eventually start to affect health in the form of chronic symptoms.

What's the usual tendency when this happens? We try and control situations even more! Eventually, we're less able to connect with how we're really feeling and the body becomes more inaccessible to us. The tools we talked about in earlier sections, such as getting at the roots of health and reading the body's signals, become more challenging to do as layers of control imprison us. The control often starts to affect our behaviors and actions in life as well. We may exercise less freedom to uniquely express ourselves or we may start feeling separate from our true natures and who we are as individuals.

---

## **Exercise:**

It can be helpful to loosen the reins at times. Do you have a daily habit or a ritual that helps you feel more in control? One that drives you a little nutty if you don't do it? Try skipping it for tomorrow. Or is there someone in your life you've been a little hard on lately? Try cutting them some slack for a day.

---

Is excessive control fair to us or to our bodies? Considering that the control isn't real and serves as more of a crutch in life, it's not fair. Much time and opportunity gets wasted when we seek to control things that are uncontrollable. By loosening the grips of this habit, we create more space for healthy changes to take place in our lives. Our thoughts and emotions are more freed up to support the things we really want to do. We also create more opportunities for enjoyment.

How much fun is control anyway?

Let's look at a case where control proved to be at the center of health disruption. A young woman named Kris, age 25, came to see me about her acne symptoms. The acne was red, inflamed, and very sensitive. Kris reported a history of digestive issues as well including alternating constipation and diarrhea, which were getting worse over time.

Kris also experienced monthly PMS with menstrual cramps and mood swings. She noticed worsening of her acne symptoms during that time. For work, Kris did different types of performance. She enjoyed her work, but even after close to three years living in the area, she still found it difficult to make friends in her field. This last point seemed to be bugging her a lot, and so we explored it a bit.

It became apparent that Kris had been feeling increased social anxiety over time. Even though she felt comfortable on stage when performing publicly, her anxieties would surface in non-performance related social situations. The anxiety grew stronger around groups of people. In fact, around the time of social events, Kris's digestive issues would flare up intensely. Kris made it a point to control her behavior so that no one could tell she was experiencing anxiety. The control she was exerting outwardly was also triggering her to suppress anxiety internally, making her feel even more anxious. Her acne got noticeably worse at these times.

During her first visit, Kris expressed a desire to get treatment for her anxiety as well. She wanted to confront these feelings rather than shove them out of the way every time they crept up. Despite her efforts to hide how she was feeling, her discomfort in groups was growing. We talked about how it's natural to experience some awkwardness and anxiety around socializing. We also touched on the fact that even though everyone else may seem more "with it" than we imagine ourselves to be in these situations, we don't know what anyone else is going through in reality. We can only focus on how we're feeling and go through any anxieties or fears that come up, so that the emotions don't get stuck and work against us.

Kris left that day with a few other natural therapies to support both her skin and anxiety, including an adaptogenic herbal formula and a homeopathic remedy. She also started on a detoxifying and balancing digestive aid that included fiber and probiotics. As her digestion became more balanced, it would help both the acne and anxiety, and vice versa. Finally, Kris switched to a gentler and more natural facial cleanser more suitable to her sensitive skin.

Kris also decided she'd like to conceal her breakouts a bit more with natural and breathable makeup, to help with outward confidence when interacting with others or her mirror. We talked about the psychology of skin issues and how the mind can become neurotic and obsessed with not only how to solve the problem, but also with the symptoms themselves. The skin can become a new area in which we try and exert control, mimicking what we're doing with the anxiety.

At each successive follow-up visit, Kris's skin looked better and better. I noticed the change in her confidence, which even influenced the dynamic of her appointments. She knew with more certainty what she wanted for her health and socially. Instead of meeting new people and instantly wondering whether they liked her, she acknowledged her own presence more during social situations.

As Kris learned how to break the habit of ignoring and suppressing herself around others in order to present a controlled persona, her digestion, anxiety, and skin symptoms calmed down, allowing her to live her life more freely. Kris's PMS symptoms improved as well as a byproduct of her connecting with her health and emotions. During this time, Kris's performance work took off in new and exciting directions that she now felt ready for.

Again, Kris didn't focus on her acne symptoms alone. If she had, she may not have seen the improvements that ended up coming into her life. She approached her full cluster of symptoms, or the "big picture" of her health, including the skin complaint, suppressed anxiety, stress, and unbalanced digestion. This inside-outside approach helped Kris learn more about herself and her health so that benefits could stick around for the long-term. Key in her ability to do this was letting go of controlling so much how she appeared to others.

---

## Challenge Questions:

*Which types of environments or situations do you try and exert control over? How might it be affecting your health?*

---

Is Kris's anxiety gone forever? Will she never get a pimple again? Those weren't the goals of her treatment. There is no such thing as a perfect life or perfect health. Health moves with the ups and downs of life, and it doesn't exist inside a bubble outside of daily living. If a particularly stressful time comes up, Kris may have increased anxiety or a flare-up of acne. That's life. During these times, however, Kris will most likely feel better able to handle what she's going through and limit the severity of symptoms and how long they last. While preparing for an important performance, Kris did in fact end up having a flare-up of acne and anxiety. Instead of panicking, Kris took care of her health and paid attention to how she was feeling. By the time the performance came, Kris's symptoms decreased and she was ready to go.

To create space for health, each of us has to accept the challenges and limitations that we realistically have to deal with while trying to be healthy. In the next section, we'll talk more about how health can't be perfect.

# NO SUCH THING AS PERFECT HEALTH

Have you ever watched a pharmaceutical commercial, in disbelief, as a once depressed individual supposedly takes their medication and feels in "perfect" and zen health every day? Or have you flipped through a health magazine and looked at "perfect" specimens of men or women posed doing yoga and weights, as if there's nothing else going on in life and they have a limitless supply of energy and smiles? Then there's a yogurt commercial where a woman drops three dress sizes and now enjoys a "perfect" figure, simply by eating more yogurt.

You'll find no shortage of messages out there that no matter what's going on in life, you should still be able to achieve perfect health. **The truth is, a perfect life and perfect health don't exist.** Trying to create health inside a perfect bubble that can't be touched is both unrealistic and unsustainable for the long-term. Every time we aim toward perfection, we end up missing the point of what health is for our own lives.

We also miss the chance to learn more about ourselves and our health on a real and meaningful level. True health isn't just superficial, it's felt throughout the body.

Each of us has limitations in both health and in life, and accepting these limitations is part of being healthy. Your life is yours. You can't have someone else's life and no one else can have your life. What this means is that each person's health is uniquely different and has to exist inside the life that person is living.

---

## Challenge Questions:

*1) When you think of your health, do you imagine a perfect picture with no symptoms, illness, negative emotions, or ups and downs?*

*2) What is a realistic view of health that is in line with your past, your experiences, your personality, and who you are overall?*

---

We regularly see examples around us of what is touted as a "perfect" diet, physique, exercise routine, sleep schedule, meditation style, or other health parameter. One question we could ask ourselves is why are we so susceptible to these images of perfection being sold by the health industry? Could it be because we are already pressuring ourselves to be perfect?

What is nefarious and rarely discussed in regards to health is the pursuit of perfection in day-to-day living. From the moment we wake up in the morning, many of us are tempted to greet ourselves with, "Good morning, how can I make today perfect?" rather than, "Hey day, let's see what happens." In the next case example, we'll explore how this mentality can be draining and makes it challenging to tap into real health.

One of my patients, Tammy, asked me during a visit, "Well, I can't quit my busy job, so aren't my symptoms going to remain unmanageable no matter what I do?" She had just looked at her hormone lab results, in which multiple deficiencies were indicating that her body was getting burnt out. Her job had come up a few times as the unchangeable and pain-in-the-butt area of her life.

Everybody has challenging and difficult situations that they have to deal with in life. Some face challenges surrounding their jobs, others around family, others around finances, and the list goes on. Life is never perfect and it has no shortage of busy, upsetting, and overwhelming moments, but amid these times it is still possible to support health in your own way.

How? When Tammy expressed her concern that her symptoms would remain unmanageable, she was forgetting one thing. Since even her first appointment, she was admitting her feelings about work more readily and not bottling them up as much. Whether it was anger, frustration, or irritation, Tammy was becoming more aware of what she was going through. In the past, she was used to maintaining the status quo with an outward appearance of having it all put together. People were used to relying on her heavily at work and at home. Tammy kept her cool and tried to have a "perfect" work persona. The more effort she was putting into being a perfect and cool worker on the outside, the more her real but suppressed reactions were affecting her body on the inside.

Meanwhile, Tammy's coworkers increasingly saw her as the perfect person to pile more responsibilities on top of, because from where they were standing, it seemed she could handle it. Less work for them! Previously, Tammy hadn't seen any connection between her emotions and her ongoing symptoms of fatigue, PMS, allergies, and acne. In fact, she had said during her first visit that she didn't experience any anger or stress and was naturally an upbeat person.

Tammy did have an upbeat side to her personality, but that wasn't who she was 100% of the time. She had other reactions to life as well which included feelings of anger and frustration. These feelings became particularly intense at work the more she tried to hide them.

Each time Tammy came in, she was more willing to talk about the connection between how she felt and her symptoms. Even more importantly, she was starting to pierce through the outward facade of perfection and was connecting with her health on a deeper level. Tammy was making it a priority to check in with herself when she felt overwhelmed or upset rather than letting it build up uncontrolled in pursuit of presenting a perfect work persona. By her third visit, Tammy's PMS symptoms had noticeably improved. She was realizing that she didn't have to hide from herself just to make things look perfect on the outside.

---

## Exercise:

Think of a recent situation in life that has been challenging, upsetting, or stressful. What has been more difficult to handle: *the situation itself, or the attempt to present a "perfect" image as if the situation doesn't affect you?* (There is no right answer to this question, but the point is that we can easily compound difficult situations when we try to appear as if they don't affect us in any way.)

Maintaining outward perfection drains energy, and that was what Tammy was feeling with her fatigue. She wanted to feel human again, both in her life and in her health. She wanted to feel like it was okay to go through difficult moments and insecurities when they came up in life.

She also craved more of an opportunity to attend to her symptoms and overall health. Tammy didn't have to quit her job to get this opportunity. Instead, she paid more attention to herself—the real person and not just the outward persona.

Each of us has a persona and certain roles that we play in life. There are work-related roles, family roles, and social roles. These roles are helpful for the settings we use them in, but at times they can threaten to overtake our true natures. Does a teacher always want to be in teacher mode? Does a mother always want to be a perfect mom? We play our roles in life, which bring out different sides of us and help us grow—but they are not all that we are. Roles can often demand a lot from us, sometimes more than we have the energy to give. If we stay true to who we are amid playing these roles, we can keep in touch with our health and personalities outside of these roles too.

When you start to feel like the role you're playing is taking over who you are, step back and ask yourself honestly whether that role is more important than you as a person. In both my own personal experiences and those of my patients, I've seen that roles can overtake life quite easily if we don't pay attention. For example, as a first time physician leaving graduate school and entering the real world, I treated "doctor" as something I had to be all the time and be perfect at in order to do the role justice. Was I aware I was doing this at first? No, because I thought it was the "norm," or something I should be doing as a naturopathic doctor.

When I let the role of "doctor" overtake life by pressuring myself to be perfect at it, ironically it didn't help me learn and grow as either a doctor or a human being. The roles we play, even when we choose them, can stifle our creativity and growth if they're all that we focus on in life. When we go back to who we are, we can still play our roles but in a more unique and enjoyable way. As part of the learning curve in my career, I started to acknowledge who I am as an individual and that being a doctor is an extension of who I am already. Many of my patients learn similar lessons as they start to take more control of their health. They will reprioritize their roles to allow more energy, creativity, and enjoyment into life. Basically, they start to put themselves first.

Where else do we have a tendency to seek perfection in life and health? Emotions. Have you ever had a bad day and instead of looking at how you're feeling, you force yourself to feel happier? You may be alone or around other people, but still the main message your brain sends is that it's not okay to feel low and that it's time to be more positive. Do you *actually feel* happier? Maybe not, but in your mind you've convinced yourself that everything's okay because at least you appear to be.

This experience happens to us all during life. As we touched on in the last two chapters, the familiar messages of "be positive" and "strive for happiness" may sound good, but it's impossible to feel this way all the time. When positivity and happiness are a part of life's highs and lows, we feel it naturally and can enjoy the moments. When we're artificially creating these feelings, however, to mask fear, sadness, anxiety, anger, depression, or frustration, we end up doing more harm than good for our health.

Maintaining an artificial high to be "on" or "perfect" actually drains the body's energy. How? When we don't attend to the real feelings that exist underneath the high, they don't get resolved. The body is designed to naturally process emotions that come up, but if we're stopping this from happening with our minds, then the feelings are driven deeper inward and the body's natural processes are disrupted. You can't trick the body into "unfeeling" something, so the neglected emotions become chronic and start to affect your health on a daily basis.

We all react to scary, upsetting, and disappointing moments in life on some level. That means that our bodies do too! The way the body feels emotions is through communication between its cells, and these messages are delivered by chemical molecules called hormones and neurotransmitters. These messengers are like mail carriers in the body.

Let's look at the biochemical communication taking place for Tammy and all of us during feelings of anger, as an example of a "negative" emotion. In response to anger, a rush of hormones and neurotransmitters (or "mail carriers") including epinephrine and norepinephrine are released inside the body. These molecules set off a burst of energy in the form of blood sugar that helps the body react to the external situation. Heart rate accelerates, blood pressure goes up, breathing becomes more rapid, and the face may flush as more blood enters the extremities in preparation for physical action. The mind becomes alert, sharp, and ready to concentrate on what's going on in the environment. Game on!

So, what happens when we squash this anger response in favor of looking peaceful or perfect on the outside—not just once but on a regular basis? The surge of energy released by the body's chemical messengers can't find a useful outlet. Instead, the whole response is turned back onto the body itself. It's almost as if by ignoring anger, we turn the anger onto ourselves rather than toward the real source of it! Over time, suppressed anger turns into chronic frustration and can start to upset the body's physiological functions, including the balance of hormones and neurotransmitters. Chronic symptoms such as fatigue, insomnia, depression, anxiety, digestive upset, allergies, acne, irritability, PMS, low libido, and many others can set in or become worse from ignoring and suppressing our anger.

---

## Exercise:

Next time you're experiencing a strong emotion, try and observe how your body physically manifests it. See if you notice reactions such as:

**Tense shoulders**
**Sweating**
**Flushing in the face**
**Cold hands**
**Chest tightness**
**Stomach queasiness**
**Rapid breathing**
**Racing heart**
**Jitteriness**

*If so, this is normal! Your body's chemical messengers are doing their jobs.*

Being aware of feelings such as anger, anxiety, or sadness helps us pay more attention to what we're going through, and we can take better care of ourselves during difficult times. If we refuse to admit when times are difficult or challenging, however, the pent up emotions continue to affect the body uninterrupted no matter what we present on the outside. Even when we're trying to act happy and positive on the outside, the inside of the body feels out of balance and distressed. The body's mail carriers become tired and the important mail gets backed up and isn't delivered efficiently to the targeted cells, leading to chronic symptoms and illness.

Suppressing what are often considered "low" or "negative" emotions in favor of a perpetual high creates a situation where the body becomes neglected too, as our suppressed anger example shows. In my opinion, denial of and detachment from these natural emotions is one of the leading causes of chronic symptoms and illness in the modern world. Societal pressure to be perfect and have it all together is immense and very real. It may seem like acting happy or positive on the outside is relieving pressure or tension in life, but it actually does just the opposite. It adds more of a burden onto our shoulders, both physically and emotionally. We all come across the challenge of acknowledging how we really feel in the face of how we supposedly *should* feel. Even if we can make everything on the surface look happy, we have to wonder where the real emotions are going and ask ourselves if this is what true health looks like.

So then, what does true health look like to you? I often tell patients to picture the changes they'd like to see in their health. The act of picturing helps us connect with our bodies, our mindset surrounding health, and our beliefs about getting healthier. In other areas of life, such as when someone wants to start a business, vision is key in getting there. Having vision about what you want helps in health too. We'll talk more about picturing health in the next section.

# PICTURING YOUR HEALTH

When chronic symptoms come up in life, it's easy for many of us to picture the last time we felt healthy and full of energy. Patients often describe to me very vividly how they *used to feel* before chronic symptoms set in, exactly how long ago that was, and what types of activities they used to do during that time. For many, it can feel like health existed in a different lifetime altogether than the present.

Though a memory of the past can remind us of our potential to feel healthy, it can also frustrate us in its discrepancy with the present. We may become so fixated on the past that picturing the return of health becomes difficult. We may also start striving for perfect future health to counteract how we're feeling today. But in reality, it's impossible to rewind time in health or flash forward in time and skip the healing process. With life's stressors and challenges, health issues can naturally arise. When they do, we can learn from them and picture what we'd like *now* for our health and our lives. **It's important to start from where you're at—in the present.**

Picturing health is a therapeutic exercise because it helps us visualize how we'd like to feel and how we'd like to look. Health is experienced both internally and externally. For example, picture those days when stress is piling up, worries and anxieties seem to be gobbling up brain cells, you end up skipping meals, and you're lacking sleep from the night before. When you glance in the mirror, can you visually see the stress? Likewise, on days when you're feeling energized and more in tune with yourself and health, the change in the mirror can be very noticeable. There may be fewer under eye circles, more hydrated and balanced skin, and a spark to your expression.

We all go through those days when we're looking at a more tired and strung out version of ourselves in the mirror, and this is normal. What you see isn't permanent. At the same time, it's helpful to notice what you're going through so you can picture better health for yourself. The mind plays a powerful role in health, as we've touched on. You can use the power of the mind to visualize how you'd like to look and feel. Picturing health works not only for external symptoms such as acne, but also for internal ones like digestive issues, anxiety, or stress.

# **Exercise:**

Try out this simple 5-10 minute visualization exercise for your health:

1. Choose a time when you're feeling relaxed, either before bed or when you're sitting in a comfortable position. Take a few deep breaths.

2. Close your eyes and do a quick scan from your head to your toes to see which areas of the body are asking for more care and attention (similar to the sensors exercise we did).

3. Remember to check in with both internal and external symptoms, including mood-related ones such as anxiety.

4. Focus on one symptom at a time. Picture your body dealing with the specific symptom at hand and imagine what you'd like to see and feel in your health.

5. Feel free to use any creative visualization techniques that your mind comes up with for each symptom. Picture health in whatever way feels natural.

During my experiences treating skin issues, I've seen the potential for the mind-body connection to make a real difference in the healing process. Picturing health is both something I talk about during health visits and write down on treatment plans.

One patient I saw for skin issues was a 21-year-old female named Daniele. This patient had a lengthy past with acne, full of frustrating moments both at home and during medical visits. Her family enjoyed poking fun at her breakouts, which made her feel self-conscious. She tried many different avenues for treatment including prescription creams at first, and then more natural options such as detoxification and cleanses, organic skincare products, and the elimination of gluten, dairy, and processed foods from her diet. The treatments produced minimal improvement, and after no time the acne would return the same or worse than before.

When I saw Daniele, she wanted to explore: What was missing? She felt in her gut that her skin could get better, but she was frustrated after having tried so many different treatments and products. It had become a familiar and painful experience to regularly search for different therapies, products, and skincare options and to keep spending money on things that didn't work. Daniele didn't know what else she could try, and she was starting to feel scared that nothing would ever work. Picturing a life with red and inflamed bumps on her face was becoming very discouraging, not just for Daniele's appearance but also her lifestyle and health in general. She instead wanted to feel like a confident young woman who could talk to other people without wondering if they noticed her skin.

It was clear that Daniele was frustrated, so we explored that feeling more. Any feeling that comes up surrounding a health issue can offer information about that symptom. As we talked, it surfaced that when Daniele thought about how she looked, her acne was always a part of that image. She had learned to picture herself with acne and it was becoming a part of her identity too. Her family made her feel worse, but even around her friends who weren't outwardly judgmental, it was hard to feel herself and this upset her. Daniele already had a predisposition to skin breakouts, but the mindset that was growing around her acne was increasing her stress and making the breakouts worse. Also, there were many feelings related to her acne that were unexplored for Daniele, and most of these feelings had been there even before the breakouts had started.

Daniele's treatment plan had a few different complementary therapies in it, but the heart of the treatment was picturing skin health. The recommendation was for Daniele to find a comfortable and relaxing position to sit in, or to do the picturing exercise before bed. Next, she could close her eyes and picture the changes she'd like to see for her health, not just for skin but also for any other symptoms she wanted improvement in. If it was challenging to relax the body and unwind the mind, we discussed muscle relaxation exercises that Daniele could do before the visualization.

The rest of the treatment plan involved a less harsh face washing routine, a homeopathic remedy, and natural hormone balancing. After a few months of hormone balancing, Daniele's menstrual cycle became more regular and she was able to discontinue that treatment. Her skin also seemed more balanced in oil production. The gentle face washing and homeopathic remedy seemed to calm the skin as well.

The key for Daniele's long-term success with reducing acne, however, was how she stuck with her visualization exercise for clearer skin. She started to notice when she felt and looked stressed, and she connected the dots that these were times when breakouts got worse. She used the picturing techniques to stay on track with managing stress and believing in her skin's health. As the months went by, Daniele's skin got used to staying mostly clear. When occasional breakouts happened, they went away in a shorter amount of time and without scarring.

The act of picturing her health how she wanted it helped Daniele *practice* clearer skin rather than falling into an extreme—of either hoping for a miracle cure or deciding that nothing would work. It also helped her have a more useful attitude toward her skin and to be more gentle toward it (and herself). We may not consciously realize it, but there can sometimes be anger and blame directed toward one's self when symptoms come up. Daniele had partly been blaming herself for not getting results with her skin and even for having acne in the first place. As Daniele's attitude opened up about her skin and her health, she was able to see more clearly the connections between acne and stress, pent-up emotions, and being overly hard on herself.

Picturing health is not a miracle cure, but the power of the mind is strong in directing how we treat ourselves and our health. Regaining health can feel challenging and sometimes discouraging. Picturing the changes we want can be a valuable tool in helping us stick with it even when times get tough.

What else can you picture for your health? Health is more than keeping the physical body strong and energized. It's also about enjoying life and finding time for activities that you like and have fun doing. The tendency when talking about health is often to be serious, earnest, rule-abiding, and sometimes militant too. The message may be that we either do it the "right way" and get rewarded in health, or if we're "bad" and don't follow the rules then our cholesterol will go up, for example. Does this sound realistic, or to some extent is it perhaps a superstitious and harsh way to think about health?

What this overly strict mentality toward health can do is suck enjoyment out of life, unnecessarily. We can still be healthy and enjoy life at the same time. Health isn't all about rules and "do's" and "don'ts." At its heart, health is sparked most when we're living our lives the way we want to and taking care of ourselves through our adventures. In the next section, we'll talk more about the relationship between health and enjoying life.

# ENJOYING LIFE IS MEDICINE

Among my patients who are sixty-five or older and keeping good health, what do you think is the one thing they all have in common? Are they taking supplements regularly, strictly watching what they eat, or hitting the gym five days a week? Do they go to the doctor for regular check-ups? Are they trying to stay happy and positive all the time?

In fact, the one thing they all have in common is that they *enjoy.* They enjoy who they are, the talents they possess, facing the challenges unique to them, the things they are learning, the things they are doing, and the way they spend their time. Difficulties still come up along the way, but the invitation for enjoyment in daily living introduces a youthful vitality for these patients, no matter what age they're at. I'll often sit across from them during visits and ask them about their favorite hobby or activity. As they're talking about what they do, patients light up and you can tell that enjoyment is as much or more a part of their health as anything they do with diet, exercise, and sleep.

Here's an example. One of my patients, Donna, came in to get some help with natural hormone balancing. She had already started treatment prior to the visit and wanted a little extra support. At her age of 65, I thought that we would spend most of the visit talking about bioidentical hormones, diet, and exercise. After ten minutes, I discovered that Donna already felt centered in her approach to health and that natural hormone balancing was just one tool she used for her overall health. I learned that Donna liked to sing in a classical choir, and that she'd been performing with this group for years. She liked both the creative element of singing and the social aspect of it within her group. As Donna talked about singing, she looked inspired and it was obvious where a big part of her balanced health was coming from.

**Achieving health doesn't always have to involve pain, suffering, and unforgiving lifestyle changes.** When we become overly militant about being healthy, this approach can actually squash natural enjoyment of life. Enjoyment is a big part of health, so it's a shame to live this way. When we stay true to who we are as unique individuals, we tend to attract healthy practices that allow us to enjoy life too.

What do you do for fun? Doctors don't often ask you this question in regards to health care, but maybe enjoyment plays more of a role in health than we openly acknowledge. Fun has great effects on both the body and mind. It gets your blood pumping, hormones and neurotransmitters flowing, gives you something to look forward to from day to day, and healthily engages your body and mind.

Sometimes when life gets stressful, there is a tendency to skip having fun because of all there is to do or think about. You might convince yourself that having a good time would be irresponsible and lead to more stress and obligations piling up. During these stressful times, your body will start hinting to you that it's time for a dose of fun. You may start to experience sluggishness, your mind may feel foggy, and your mood may throw more anxiety and irritability your way. You might feel just generally out of balance.

What your body is telling you is that it's time to shake things up a bit and distract yourself from the stress and worries. What is fun? These days, fun may conjure up images of watching videos online, playing on a tablet or smart phone, and catching up with social media. While these all can be enjoyable in moderation, it can also be helpful to step away from the screens temporarily to try out other types of fun.

Think about how you feel after spending a weekend doing something that interests you. Fun and enjoyment are sparked by activities that tap into who you are and help bring out your natural talents and personality. It can involve challenges and learning, such as writing a creative story or picking up a new instrument. It can also involve more frivolous activities like playing frisbee outside, going for a hike, seeing a new movie, or beating a friend at Battleship. While these activities may seem obvious, they're some of the first ones we can neglect when stress enters the picture. Having fun helps you grow, learn new things about yourself, and stretch your imagination.

---

# Exercise:

Even though doctors don't ask how much fun you have, it's a good idea to ask yourself once in a while. Is there an activity that you enjoy that you haven't had a chance to do much lately? If so, rearrange your schedule a bit or write a reminder on a Post-it note so that you hold yourself to getting back to it. See if a friend wants to join you if you think that would be fun. And for extra fun, ditch the screens for a day.

---

You'll most likely find that after having a good time, the daunting nature of stress, work, and other responsibilities softens around the edges. You'll feel renewed energy for dealing with the challenges that are on your plate and any others that might pop up. And you can say to yourself, "Hey—I had fun and feel better. I deserve it!"

Sometimes when we think about having fun, the police officer in our minds can take over and say it's not allowed because problems in life haven't been solved yet. Life has a never ending supply of what can be labeled as problems. If we wait for the problems to end, we don't get a chance to enjoy ourselves enough. The point of life isn't to stay in constant alert for impending danger and problems. Those people who are still doing what they enjoy later on in life, allowing themselves doses of fun, and staying healthy are good examples that life is about a whole lot more than that.

What can happen when we're constantly alert for things going wrong in life? The body can actually become stuck in a state of waiting for that danger to come, and other physiological processes can get thrown off in the meantime. This state of hypersensitivity can lead to autoimmune symptoms and conditions. What is autoimmunity? We'll take a look at this topic closely in the next section.

# AUTOIMMUNITY TODAY

Autoimmunity is growing at an alarming rate in today's world. Conditions such as allergies, eczema, thyroid disorders, and food sensitivities are more widespread now than ever before. Kids as young as toddlers, or even infants, can develop eczema and continue to have flares well into adulthood. What's going on? Why are these types of health issues becoming so common?

Normally, the immune system only attacks what it sees as a "foreign invader," such as bacteria, viruses, and other germs. In autoimmunity, the body starts attacking its own cells and can no longer distinguish what is friend versus foe in its internal environment. Autoimmunity weakens and confuses the immune system's functioning, and this can often snowball, leading to even more autoimmune symptoms. What can we do to throw some water on this fire?

**It's important to realize that autoimmunity is not simply an internal phenomenon, but that its**

**initial triggers frequently stem from reactions we have to our external environments.** In other words, the mind is also involved. We are each distinct individuals, but we also exist as part of the environments we spend time in. Naturally, we have responses to these environments and the people we interact with in them. The responses we have can affect how we feel in our health.

These days, it is hard to deny that the popularity of the internet and social media has created a technologically oriented culture where social boundaries have become more blurred. When anything and everything can somehow end up on cyberspace or be tapped into by the net, we all feel more watched and scrutinized by others. As a backlash to dwindling privacy for the individual, society has become increasingly more censored and politically correct.

"What's the right thing to say, and what's the right way to act?" we may find ourselves wondering more often. As a result, we are more hypersensitive to our own and other's behaviors and find it challenging to distinguish between friend or foe in the outside world. Sound familiar?! When we feel hypersensitive in our environments, always trying to protect ourselves from those who might do us harm or from something going "wrong," this hypersensitivity can exert strong effects on the body as well.

> # **Challenge Questions:**
>
> *When was the last time you questioned yourself on whether you were acting the "right" way? How did you feel in that moment?*

As occurs a lot in health, the microcosm often reflects the macrocosm. In our daily lives, we can end up feeling torn about who to trust around us and a very strong, but overly protective instinct can set in. Physiologically, our high levels of social alertness and vigilance can induce a state of confusion and hypersensitivity in the body as well. **What is autoimmunity at its core?** It involves an overly protective immune system that has gone somewhat haywire and can no longer discern what to trust in the body versus what to attack. In the end, "self" is attacked when it shouldn't be.

I find that many of my patients are innately aware of a social and autoimmune connection in their health. Patients have frequently described to me how their autoimmune symptoms and allergies tend to flare up worse during overwhelming, uncertain, or confusing social situations. In the privacy of my office they feel comfortable talking about this connection, but I often learn that when these experiences come up in patients' daily lives, they feel pressured to act like "everything's normal." While trying to act like nothing is affecting them, patients' symptoms tend to get worse. This phenomenon rings true for many of us regardless of the specific symptoms we're going through.

There may not yet be a scientific explanation to fully account for this effect, but the connection is an important one to explore in health today. There are a couple areas to consider in the body.

Cortisol levels may be involved here to some extent. How? When we feel more guarded, the body tenses up and stress builds, depleting cortisol levels. Normally, cortisol helps balance the immune system and makes sure that inflammation and other protective immune functions don't get out of hand. If cortisol dips too low from the constant stress of perceived dangers in our environments, inflammation may be left unchecked and the immune system can start to exert effects beyond its usual boundaries.

Also, perpetual alarm that we may feel within our environments allows the *sympathetic* branch of the nervous system to dominate over the *parasympathetic* branch. Sympathetic responses of the nervous system, whether from imagined or real circumstances, are related to fight-or-flight actions. When we see imminent danger, our bodies naturally choose to either flee or stand ground and prepare for battle. The parasympathetic branch has an opposite effect of relaxing the body and supporting more leisurely processes such as digestion and sleep. When there is a chronic dominance of the sympathetic branch, we never get to rest because we're always alert for what might go wrong around us. Experiencing our surroundings in this acute way makes us more hypersensitive to what is happening externally and wears down our nervous system, and over time we become less tuned in to our own bodies and minds. This state has a parallel effect on the immune system, and in fact many autoimmune conditions do affect the nervous system in some way.

It's interesting that blurred or hypersensitive boundaries with our external environments can create blurred boundaries in our defensive (immune) systems too. Trying to distinguish between friend and foe on a regular basis can put us in a perpetual defensive stance in life. This level of guardedness also compromises processes such as sleep and digestion that need rest and relaxation for optimal function. Even though it may seem in the moment that the defensive position is protecting us, maybe it's actually putting us in more danger at times. If we're constantly on the lookout for danger, we're essentially putting ourselves in a cage and restricting our natural movement through life.

Inhibiting our natural life force through overprotection doesn't support the body, and it doesn't allow the body to feel naturally strong or resilient like it's built to be. What may seem like protection can actually make us feel stuck in place, paralyzed, and more vulnerable to our environments.

Environmental connections to autoimmunity can be easy to miss unless you take a step back and look at them more closely. A 34-year-old male patient named Dan came to see me for chronic allergic symptoms, including sneezing, congestion, runny nose, and itchy eyes. The allergies had been going on since he was a teenager, and they were unresponsive to over-the-counter allergy medications. When Dan got hit with an onslaught of allergies, he would get extremely tired and his body felt like shutting down to the world. In fact, the only thing that helped Dan feel better was sitting quietly by himself.

I asked Dan if he'd ever had a break from his allergies, and he replied that he had after moving from his hometown to California two years prior. He assumed that the change of natural habitat had helped calm his allergies down and was surprised to be revisited by them so suddenly. I asked Dan if anything had changed in his life recently, and he talked about how his wife was pregnant and he was going to be a first time dad. He was very happy about this change, but his family had been in touch with him more often since the news. Family introduced an element of stress into Dan's life that could be overwhelming, and Dan realized that his worst symptoms were occurring around those family phone calls. In fact, the first time Dan had ever experienced relief from his symptoms had been after moving farther away from his family.

Dan's family could be supportive, caring, and giving in how they interacted with him, but this wasn't the whole story. They also had a history of behaving in a direct opposite manner that felt critical, neglectful, and belittling. Just because Dan was now an adult of 34 years, didn't mean the dynamic had become more straightforward and trustworthy over time. Since Dan had a hard time distinguishing whether his family was friend or foe in his external life, the same dynamic extended to his immune system on the inside. When his family was in touch, Dan's immune system developed a blurred boundary surrounding what to trust in the body versus what to guard against. This effect brought on severe and hypersensitive allergic responses.

Dan knew he would continue to hear from his family. Very often, we're not able to change the environment that we're dealing with. However, we can change how we react to situations and the mindset we have while in the environment. Dan wanted to have more privacy again so he and his wife could enjoy the pregnancy and look forward to new changes. The added family stress was getting in the way of the enjoyment, so Dan decided to set his own boundaries instead of allowing family members to dictate what they were going to be.

He was also more honest with himself when symptoms flared as to what might be triggering them. Doing so helped Dan to take a step back from stressful situations so he could attend more to himself and his health. Adding in an immunomodulator, good water intake, and more rest, Dan's allergy flares gradually improved until they were infrequent and shorter in duration.

During his journey with health, Dan also learned about how his personality played a part in his symptoms, which we explored during his homeopathy intake. When Dan was younger, he was an extremely open kid and he would let his bubbly personality out more often. He was also more trusting of his environment and wasn't in the habit of holding his guard up. As he entered his teenage years and experienced more hurtful and confusing situations with his family and out in the world, his natural tendencies started to change and he grew more sensitive to his environment and other people's reactions. This increased sensitivity led Dan to put his guard up more often and to feel over-protective. Dan realized that he missed the openness he used to feel when he was younger, and which he felt was more true to his personality.

Dan felt that guarding himself so tightly wasn't helping him get through allergies, and in fact the habit was making him feel closed off and worsening his symptoms. As he tensed up in different environments, his personality wasn't allowed to come out and the avoidance of "trouble" or "danger" was making him feel hypersensitive to what could happen. It seemed like the hypersensitivity he felt was spreading to his immune system too.

It can be challenging to admit how an environment affects you, your health, and your personality. In the moment, it can appear as if everyone else is doing fine and is unaffected, so we convince ourselves that we should feel that way too. There can be a lot of pressure to fit in and not stand out in a crowd, and as we've discussed, there is a tendency to hold real emotions in check so that there's less risk of others noticing them. We're all susceptible in our own ways to peer pressure to fit in, follow social norms, and hide our real reactions.

No matter how we *decide* to react to a situation, the body has its own natural response to environments and social interactions. The signals that it sends out in the form of symptoms alert us when it's time to try a new approach. Especially in the case of allergies, eczema, food sensitivities, thyroid-related symptoms, or other autoimmune conditions, it's helpful to be aware of hypersensitive and overly defensive reactions we have to our surroundings. When we are constantly preparing and bracing ourselves for the worst, the body stays alert and can't relax. The immune system can't relax either and it easily becomes reactive to the smallest trigger, even at the risk of attacking the body itself.

If we want our immune systems to be more targeted and discerning, we can pay more attention to when we feel overstimulated in life. As we talked about earlier, the microcosm often reflects the macrocosm. In this day and age, especially with the rise in popularity of the internet and social media, disconnect from personality and the body is more common and it's even more important to recognize when the body and mind feel overwhelmed by excessive stimuli.

But it's not just technology. As we learned from Dan's example, it's challenging to admit when supposedly caring and "benevolent" stimulus (in the case of his family) can also carry more harmful properties. Doing so can bring up guilt, but approaching social stimuli in a more honest way can also help reduce hypersensitivity in our lives and in our health.

On a larger scale, overall trust in our society is quite low and perhaps this mistrust also correlates with the high occurrence of autoimmune disease these days. We want to be able to trust in others, but it's not always possible in the idealistic way we sometimes envision it. While symptoms such as eczema or allergies can feel so annoying in the moment, they are actually helpful communicators that it's time to take a more realistic view of the effects the environment can have on our health.

There is another way in which the body's health can become overwhelmed and over-stimulated: when we focus nonstop on symptoms. Throughout this book, we've talked about how it's important to pay attention to the body and notice the signals that it sends us. Paying attention to symptoms is different, however, than obsessing about them. Often, when symptoms arise there is a tendency to overly focus on them and worry to the point that we make ourselves feel worse in the process. In the next section, we'll talk more about giving symptoms the space they need to heal.

# AVOID FIXATING ON SYMPTOMS

There is a tendency in health care to want immediate results when symptoms arise. The medical community does little to alleviate this outlook with its claims that pharmaceuticals can immediately fix health problems. **Chronic health complaints have shown over time, however, to be very resistant to "instant fixes," as many people are familiar with.** We're all susceptible to the quick fix mentality and at times it can cause us to obsess over symptoms, with the hope that we can make illness magically disappear. Symptoms seldom just disappear, and we can end up caught in a cycle of stressing over them, excessively focusing on them, and even attacking them mentally or with harsh treatments to try and destroy them.

It's important to pay attention to the body, but doing so in a forceful, critical, and neurotic way in order to try and will away symptoms doesn't help. There is a strong tendency toward this behavior in health care, and I've noticed this both in my own health and that of my patients. What is the best way to break this cycle and strike a more balanced approach to health? One of my patients demonstrated this balance well and she discovered it by actively working to change her attitude and mindset surrounding health. She went above and beyond what was discussed during her naturopathic visit and kept developing her detective skills at home regarding her symptoms.

Ella was a 25-year-old graduate student with chronic acne that had started during her teens. The acne consisted of large cysts around her jaw and cheeks that refused to heal. When working with patients who are experiencing skin issues, often I'll ask how the symptoms make them feel. It was clear that Ella was very frustrated and almost choked up about her skin.

It felt to Ella like her skin symptoms had always made life stressful on top of the challenges she was already dealing with. They never seemed to give her a break and she never knew when and why they would flare up. Each day seemed structured around her "bumps," as Ella called them, and the chronic habit of tracking them created a roller coaster of emotions for her. She felt superstitious about the acne, thinking that she must be doing something "wrong" whenever the symptoms got worse.

The neurosis Ella felt about her acne translated

into the way she treated her skin too. She had not liked her skin since before she hit her teenage years. With a distaste toward her symptoms, Ella had a tendency to pick at her pimples, attack them with harsh products, and obsess over them. She also cleansed her skin only briefly with medicated washes that seemed to dry the surface out. Ella's harsh and impatient skin care routine, combined with the stress that the acne made her feel, seemed to cause even more breakouts.

---

### **Challenge Questions:**

*What symptom, or symptoms, do you have a tendency to fixate on? How has this habit affected your health?*

---

I started Ella on a gentler face wash that wouldn't strip the natural oils from her skin and cause excess sebum production (which can frequently lead to increased acne). We also worked on natural hormone balancing for Ella since she had symptoms related to her menstrual cycle clustering with the acne. As we discussed earlier, an important component of her getting well was picturing her skin feeling clear and developing a mind-body connection with her skin. What should she pay attention to? Namely, her feelings towards her skin and any stress that may be contributing to the breakouts.

Ella took her plan seriously, and within weeks she saw calmer skin from the gentler wash and reduced menstrual acne flare-ups from the hormone balancing. Ella's face was noticeably starting to clear up, but at some point she hit a plateau and didn't see much increased progress. At first, she asked me whether there was anything else she could take for the acne symptoms to improve even further. I explained how the journey to improved skin can take time and that she was doing well. Her graduate school exams were coming up, however, so Ella felt frustrated that her skin might regress and get worse again.

I offered one other skin care product for Ella to try in a pinch, but she didn't follow up on purchasing it. Instead, Ella decided on her own to revisit her health roots in relation to her skin. She decided not to panic, and instead took a step back from her situation and remembered what she had expressed to me during her visit. Obsessing over her acne made her skin feel worse. Instead of focusing on exams, she was focusing more on her acne symptoms and was trying to "figure out" a perfect and quick solution to the problem. Ella decided to try a different approach for a change.

Ella took a break to relax and do some picturing exercises for her skin like we had covered during her visit. She acknowledged to herself the feelings she was having toward her skin, including an overwhelming fixation on them. After her visualization, she decided to pay as little attention to her skin as possible except for light washing. For the next few days, Ella hardly had to deal with her acne at all. Usually within the day, and sometimes within hours, the pimples would calm down on their own without her constant attention to them. Ella's new approach was working to calm down not only her mind, but also her skin.

Pleased with the results, Ella kept practicing these techniques every time acne surfaced. She would especially take care not to fixate too much on her symptoms. Notice that she did not ignore the acne with the hopes that it would go away. Instead, she acknowledged the symptoms as well as her underlying feelings toward them rather than overly obsessing and focusing on the symptoms.

After a few months, Ella's skin was smooth and she would only have an occasional breakout rather than daily occurrences. Ella was amazed that *she herself* had created this improvement in her skin, better than any product could do. At the same time, she knew she had it in her to be a true detective into her acne symptoms. At Ella's next couple of visits, I took note that her old acne scars were visibly healing now that her breakouts were infrequent. Ella's clear skin made her shine even more, and she was enjoying the feeling it brought to her life. Even better, she did it!

Ella learned a valuable lesson that we can all benefit from in health and in life: **Fixating on a problem doesn't always make it better.** Sometimes, if we let the problem exist without looking for an immediate solution, it can actually get better naturally. Like we've talked about in previous sections, the mind is a powerful tool and we can use it in different ways for health care. A "quick fix" mentality often shortchanges the body's true potential for natural healing. When we allow the mind to connect with the symptoms we're experiencing, we can better support and harness the body's innate healing ability.

Health-related stress can come not only from fixation on symptoms, but also from focusing too much on possible "dangers" out there in the world. The main buzz words these days include: toxins, pollutants, allergens, irritants, chemicals, preservatives, additives, certain foods and the list goes on, with new ones invented all the time. While it's true that each of us can benefit from fresh air and as little toxicity as possible, we all live in a world that is both man-made as well as part of nature. Living with a constant fear of toxins can limit not only enjoyment of life, but also the potential for health. We'll explore this topic more in the next section.

# TOXINS, POLLUTANTS, AND ALLERGENS, OH MY!

Frequently, patients who come see me for their first visit are tangled in a list of things they're trying to avoid on a daily basis. They could have learned about the forbidden items in a health magazine, from the news, from another practitioner, or from a friend. Essentially, the list of what not to do can get so long that there are few items remaining on the "okay" list at the end of the day.

Impure water and air, gluten, dairy, sugar, dust, pollen, xenoestrogens, GMO products, processed foods, refined flour, foods that aren't organic, foods unbalanced in pH, food sensitivities, caffeine, unnatural cleaning products and laundry detergents, non-environmentally conscious makeup and cosmetics, and more. *Phew!* After patients have restructured their lives to stay away from these offenders, they are often surprised to see they don't feel much better and are experiencing more anxiety than before regarding day to day life. **They start to wonder, "What *is* allowed?"**

Stubborn conditions such as chronic fatigue syndrome and fibromyalgia are difficult to treat with traditional medicine, so many people turn to natural health for relief. On the natural health side, however, there is often an overly pronounced focus on identifying "offenders" such as toxins, allergens, and pollutants that are causing symptoms. But what is a toxin? And if a nutritionist tells you that you're sensitive to all fruit, is that a good enough reason to cut fruit entirely out of your diet?

I've had patients who have experienced degrees of improvement in their symptoms from changed habits such as cutting back on gluten and dairy, or avoiding processed foods. Still, patients come in for more help because they didn't experience a full resolution of symptoms and the gluten, for example, wasn't the ultimate culprit in how they were feeling. It often turns out to be just a trigger for symptoms instead, one that is indicative of a preexisting imbalance in the health of one or more of the body's systems.

**We have to ask ourselves whether we sometimes over-vilify substances in the  environment instead of taking a closer look at why we're more susceptible to these triggers in the first place.** Strengthening the body and its organ systems often proves to be more helpful for long-term health than relying on long lists of "things not to do." Policing life in this manner, especially when it's not improving symptoms, can make us very guarded toward and suspicious of our environments in general. This censorship can make it difficult for us to relax and enjoy life, which can ultimately be a downside for health rather than a truly preventive or healthy measure.

One of my patients, a 35-year-old woman named Vicky, had chronic allergies and had visited a number of providers to investigate why. She saw a nutritionist, a functional medicine provider, a naturopath, and a couple of other health practitioners. When Vicky came to see me, she was armed with the summaries and reports they had all provided her. Every report emphasized something she should stay away from. A food sensitivity panel advised her to stay away from all fruit, olives, and tomatoes. With Vicky's Mediterranean cultural background and its typical diet, she was devastated to hear she could no longer eat olives or tomatoes. The panel also advised her to avoid wheat combined with sugar in any meal.

In addition to the food sensitivity panel, we went through three other reports that admonished Vicky's current habits and environmental influences. The list of things Vicky should look out for included everything from heavy metal toxicity to watermelons. Vicky felt more confused than ever on where to start for improving her allergies. As we talked more about Vicky's previous health recommendations, she mentioned that she felt no personal connection to them. She expressed frustration that unless she could relate with health advice, it was typically hard for her to follow through with it. Vicky had tried one week of staying away from olives and tomatoes and couldn't eat half of her usual diet, which was a pretty healthy one to begin with.

Though Vicky's other providers had done tests and given her reports to clarify her condition for her, ironically Vicky couldn't think clearly about her own health after reviewing them. She was scared to do anything, for fear that it would make her symptoms worse. As Vicky talked, I noticed her stress start to increase while just listing out the things she could no longer eat or do. So for Vicky, we started treatment with a blank slate. If she wanted to eat olives and tomatoes as part of her traditional diet, she could definitely continue doing that. If she wanted to eat a pastry once in a while that combined wheat and sugar, that was fine for her to enjoy too. And she could eat fruit if she enjoyed it. We talked about how these supposed "criminals" were likely not causing her allergy symptoms directly.

After discussing Vicky's stress and energy levels,

it became clear that adrenal imbalance was throwing off her immune system and causing her body to react more strongly to environmental factors such as pollen and dust. Since pollen and dust are everywhere and are therefore unavoidable, the key wasn't to build a giant plastic bubble for her to live inside of, but instead to help Vicky's adrenal glands recover. Vicky was also tired much of the time, so we discussed strategies to help her strengthen and refuel her body, including getting away from her computer more often to go outside and exercise. It turned out that high levels of anxiety were adding to Vicky's worn-down adrenals, so we talked about how to work through those emotions.

Vicky kept eating fruit, olives, and tomatoes and still experienced improvement in her allergy symptoms after strengthening her body and organ systems. The reduction of unnecessary policing in her life gave her more freedom to live the way she wanted to. She didn't have to worry about every little thing she did, and the energy that was freed up as a result could be turned toward more helpful health measures. As an added benefit of working on her allergies, Vicky also experienced relief for her anxiety levels. She decided on her own to cut back on gluten and dairy (but not entirely eliminate them) because it made her feel better overall, not because it was what she was supposed to do. Because Vicky stuck to treatments that made sense to her and to her body, she not only improved her main symptom of allergies, but also strengthened her overall health.

There is nothing wrong with paying attention to the health of our environments, the air we surround ourselves with, and the quality of what we put into our bodies. In fact, a moderate regard of these practices can be very good for health. Some of my patients benefit from watching how much gluten and dairy they eat, for example, especially when they're healing from digestive complaints, allergies, fatigue, weight issues, skin conditions, and autoimmune symptoms.

What is helpful to be aware of, however, is going overboard with avoidance strategies—especially when they don't make sense on an individual level or are causing needless anxieties. This approach neglects to address the potential underlying causes in the body or in life that are leaving you predisposed to the offending factors. Also, if you're in the habit of questioning every morsel of food you eat, there's a possibility that you're creating more stress than you need to and unintentionally overriding your body's natural healing abilities.

When deciding which steps to take for avoiding certain foods or lifestyle influences, ask yourself whether the changes feel realistic and sustainable for you. Can you imagine staying on the new routine for three months, six months, a year, or the rest of your life without adding more stress to your days? If you're unsure, you may be able to tell after a two- or three-month trial how willing your body and mind are to stay on track. If you find that the change is difficult and disrupts life in a way you're not comfortable with, it's okay to take a different approach.

---

## Challenge Question:

*How has avoidance impacted your health? Try and weigh the pros and cons of the avoidance habits you've put in place.*

---

Lifestyle changes don't have to be all or nothing. In the case of Vicky, she didn't cut gluten and dairy completely out of her diet, but instead found benefits from simply cutting back on the higher amounts she was used to consuming. By doing so, she diversified her diet and tried out new types of foods.

In the next section, we'll talk more about why the body often resists all-or-nothing approaches to health in general. In today's culture, both in and out of medicine, quick changes seem to be favored over gradual, steady, and reasonable ones. We're bombarded by messages of which consumer goods, lifestyle measures, exercise programs, diets, and outlook adjustments will make us feel new and improved in who we are overnight:

Want to lose weight? "Just follow these seven steps!"

Tired of acne? "No problem—take this one product!"

Feeling low? "That's okay, just think positive thoughts!"

Feel insecure? "Just buy this new car!"

Around every corner, there seems to be a quick answer for every issue in life. Yet, as we've discussed, the body and mind don't operate well on instant fixes or overnight transformations. Let's explore further why this is the case, starting with a simple and cool concept called *homeostasis.*

# HOMEOSTASIS: THE BODY'S TEETER-TOTTER

Believe it or not, the body wants to keep its internal environment as unexciting as possible while it adapts to changing circumstances. In other words, it doesn't seek or support drastic changes in how it functions. The body strives for what is called *homeostasis,* which is a basic balance or equilibrium in the internal environment. It resists big shifts, regardless of whether they are positive or negative in nature. What is homeostasis in a nutshell?

Homeostasis is the body's internal teeter-totter. Think back to when you last played on a teeter-totter at a playground. A teeter-totter has a center point and moves up and down on either side of it. Imagine you and your friend are taking turns going up and down. All of a sudden, your friend is at the bottom and decides to get off quickly. What happens to you? You thud down to the ground on the opposite side, in what can be a painful fashion. There are times for big changes in life, but as far as the body's concerned, it likes to meet with change at a manageable pace if possible. It prefers slight movements of its teeter-totter rather than big and sudden ones. This is the body's safeguard against extremes and imbalances in health.

Think about if you had to jump from kindergarten all the way to college and were expected to keep up with the work. Even though you'd be learning, which is a positive influence, the changes would be way too quick and unreasonable for you to adjust to. The body also doesn't want to go from kindergarten all the way to college, metaphorically speaking. **It likes realistic and reasonable portions of change.** Even when we're trying to get healthier, it's a good idea to respect the body's natural rhythm when trying to make healthy changes.

My patients tend to acknowledge that "magic bullet" fixes in health care, such as pharmaceutical drugs or the latest health fad, are not by themselves the best tools for living a long and healthy life. But just because people understand this concept doesn't mean they're automatically swayed away from other quick fixes or the desire for overnight transformations in health. We've all dealt with the frustration of wanting a problem to disappear instantaneously, whether it's health-related or related to some other area of life.

Even though it's common to feel this way, in health this desire can lead to yo-yo dieting, extreme health habits, inconsistency in taking care of oneself, overreliance on outside authorities, and a lack of real progress in getting healthier.

Why does the body enforce homeostasis and resist our more ambitious efforts even when we're trying to get healthier? Wouldn't it be a good thing if the body experienced speedy recovery toward health, rather than having to deal with regular and persistent symptoms and health issues?

For one, many ongoing symptoms and health complaints that people experience on a daily basis aren't born overnight, or "acutely." Examples of *acute health issues* include a cold, flu, or cut. When you have one of these acute health problems, it usually takes a few days to a couple of weeks at most to get over the symptoms. The contributing factor to a common cold is simple—it's a virus (although to be fair the strength of a person's immune system and overall health will play a part in determining how long it takes to get over the cold). The body's immune system can usually get over the virus with a little help from rest, fluids, and vitamin C. These acute symptoms are quick to arise and fairly quick to resolve.

*Chronic health issues,* on the other hand, often have multiple factors underlying them and the symptoms take a lot more time to set in. Chronic symptoms also tend to have a cumulative or snowball effect on the body. They can take root over months or years, and the seeds forming them are often in place well before we detect noticeable symptoms on the outside. The effects of ongoing stress, neglected health and lifestyle, and suppressed feelings often simmer under the surface for a while before patients report actual symptoms such as insomnia or chronic fatigue. Once the symptoms do appear, they tend to reflect disruption in other organ systems in the body too, which can potentially lead to even more symptoms.

So, if chronic symptoms make their home in the body *over time*, how can we expect them to disappear *overnight*? If there are multiple underlying factors leading to chronic health issues, how can we force them all to change with a snap of the fingers? The truth is, the more we're able to deal with the roots of our health issues, the better we can help the body overcome chronic conditions in a way that works with our unique physiology rather than against it.

Pharmaceutical drugs are not the only magic bullet approaches to health care. Trying to force the body to return once again to a state of health that it may not have felt for a while through extreme diet or exercise practices, overreliance on supplements, or mental fear tactics actually makes up another form of "magic bullet" treatment. Our own mindsets can get caught up in the illusion that the body should recover overnight, regardless of whether we follow conventional or natural systems of health care. Since you are the most important coach toward better health in your life, it's helpful to learn how to realistically support the body's natural healing potential.

How can you work with the body's desire for homeostasis in your health efforts? Two subtle shifts in your mindset can help tremendously: 1) Weave patience into what you do, and 2) Resist the urge to emerge "new and improved" from your health routines. You are you, and just because you're trying to get healthier doesn't mean you have to be a completely different person to achieve it. You can regain health being exactly who you are. We can all benefit from learning about ourselves along the way, but the "new and improved" approach, in addition to being unrealistic, can lead to feelings of deficiency rather than a renewed confidence toward better health.

Also, just because you're patient with yourself in your efforts doesn't mean that you're not taking your health seriously. There is often a tendency, for example, to look at people who spend 1-2 hours a day at the gym seven days a week, and assume that health efforts always have to look like that. Patience, however, has tremendous therapeutic value and there's no need to jump hurriedly toward someone else's lifestyle just because it looks correct in theory. You're living within your body and in your lifestyle, not another person's. It's okay to be gentle and caring toward yourself as you work toward what you want in your health . Try to take on realistic changes that make sense for you rather than striving for drastic results. Patience will support your body's homeostasis and help health efforts be more consistent and effective for the long-term.

Let's take a look at a case example to demonstrate the setbacks that are possible from yo-yo or extreme health habits. A 28-year-old male named Justin came to see me for help with weight loss. Two years prior, he had lost 30 pounds all at once through an intense cleanse, hours of exercise, and a very strict diet. Justin was happy at that time to reach his weight goals and expected the results to stick around for the long-term. He then moved to the Bay Area and entered a new field of work, one that demanded long hours. All of a sudden, Justin's weight started creeping back up until he had regained all 30 pounds and 10 more pounds on top of that.

Justin was frustrated when he came to see me, and he also felt that he'd failed himself by gaining all the weight back that he had worked so hard to lose. He also feared that with his new busy schedule, it would prove difficult to follow the same steps he'd taken two years prior to lose weight. Because he had lost weight quickly before, however, he expected the same changes to happen again. He decided that stringent health measures were the only way to go, but he was having a harder time sticking to them this time around.

Justin's tone throughout our conversation was one of wanting to feel new and improved again, like he had two years ago after losing 30 pounds. It was as if he believed there was a magic button somewhere out there to push, and if he could just find it the weight would come off automatically. Justin was getting more and more frustrated seeking this button and he wasn't able to see this frustration clearly. He felt the frustration was coming from his weight issues, while his "new and improved" mindset surrounding health was actually upsetting him more.

After completing a men's health questionnaire, we were able to connect the dots that Justin's hormones were out of balance from a surge of increased stress over the previous year. His relocation to a new area combined with a new and demanding job were both contributing to adrenal fatigue in his body. Labs showed that both testosterone and cortisol hormone levels were low, leading to low energy and mood. The hormone deficiencies were slowing down Justin's metabolism, creating more sluggishness in the body rather than efficient use of fuel (both from meals and fat stores).

Justin admitted to having low energy, and he felt that it was decreasing his motivation to exercise and keep up with his health. He also shared that he demanded a lot from himself and his health goals and that he would often skip exercise altogether rather than face the guilt of not doing enough. In other words, when he couldn't put in at least one intense hour at the gym, Justin chose to forego even something simple like a walk for exercise. He had very little patience toward himself, and he tended to put himself down regularly without realizing it.

Additionally, multiple symptoms were creeping up along with his weight that were creating more obstacles to weight loss. Justin faced sleep issues, constant sugar and carbohydrate cravings, and anxiety combined with depression. Again, Justin's habits surrounding these symptoms were all-or-nothing. For example, if he couldn't stick to a gluten-free diet 100% of the time, he would overindulge in sugar and carbohydrates instead. This behavior was strongly tied to his desire for a fast "magic bullet" solution.

Justin and I discussed a treatment plan that would be more realistic for his current schedule, and he contributed to it with his ideas. It included an adaptogen for stress relief and natural medicine for raising testosterone levels. It also included reasonable steps for balancing diet, exercise, and sleep habits. The core of Justin's treatment plan as a whole encouraged him to be less hard on himself. The less mired he felt in a cycle of guilt, the more potential he'd have to make real changes in his health and weight. The goal was not to shed 30 pounds overnight, but instead to strengthen and balance the whole body's health so that weight loss could come about more naturally over time.

During Justin's follow-up visits, however, he was resistant to reasonable weight loss steps and instead kept his all-or-nothing approach. Despite what we had come up with at his first visit, smaller steps didn't seem good enough for him. He would try them for a bit and feel good, but when stress got high he tended to be harder on himself and his body. At that time, he would start chastising himself for not going to the gym more regularly and not staying gluten and sugar free. Ironically, his self-blame led to the opposite habits of skipping exercise altogether and eating gluten and sugar in excess.

After a period of guilt, Justin would forget about the more realistic treatment plan he had started and felt improvement from. He would force himself to cut out all gluten, sugar, and dairy and go to the gym every day. After a month of consistent efforts, he would experience some weight loss but also felt too tired to continue. At that point, he would gain all the weight back again. **Justin was having to recover from his yo-yo habits even more so than from his actual symptoms.** He was also exacerbating his body's adrenal fatigue state.

---

# Exercise:

Think about your current health habits and pinpoint which ones haven't been bringing about the changes you want to see. Especially highlight those habits which have felt inconsistent. Write each of these habits out and next to them, brainstorm ways to make these approaches more doable, reasonable, and potentially more effective.

---

At that point in time, Justin was not yet in a place where he was willing to be more flexible in his approach to his weight and overall health. He was in a position of being hard on himself, and most likely he had been doing that for a while. The way he treated himself made it challenging for him to really look at the underlying connections in health that were leading to weight gain in the first place. Instead he wanted quick and guaranteed solutions, ones that would supposedly transform him into a new and improved person. Justin now had tools available that could help him feel better health in line with his body's physiology, but he wasn't ready to use them yet. He'd first have to explore the amount of pressure he put on himself on a daily basis that was blocking his road to health.

In this example, Justin chose natural approaches to weight loss, which perhaps wouldn't normally be considered "magic bullet" treatments. However, his mindset was geared toward finding an instant fix and for that reason, even the natural methods he employed worked against the homeostasis of his body. When we're seeking health, there will be some resistance to change in the body because of the mechanism of homeostasis. We can work with the body and its natural rhythm better if we are patient and avoid the promises offered by quick solutions. The body needs time to adjust to treatment, especially in the case of chronic conditions.

Homeostasis doesn't only apply to the physical body, but also to our minds. We each have patterns that develop over time related to the way that we think about our health, how we see ourselves, and how we view change. These established ways of thinking influence our habits and the decisions we make toward health, or any other area of life, on a daily basis. When we try and order the mind to wrap itself around an extreme health routine or change of mindset without considering where it's realistically at, we're working against ourselves. The mind will naturally resist this approach to health in the same way the body does.

Think about the amount of time it probably took Justin to adjust to a new area and job situation. The body and mind are the same, in that they need time to adapt to changing circumstances and routines. Starting from where you're at will help you work with homeostasis. When you give yourself time and space to adjust instead of forcing change upon your life, there is better potential for long-term health and vitality.

As we touched on in the introduction and in this example, personality does play a part in health. Our personalities shape how we live our lives and health is tied directly to lifestyle. Getting in touch with our unique personalities can give us insight into where our strengths lie in health, areas we need to work on, our fears and anxieties surrounding health, and how we might be creating our own obstacles to better health. The next section will talk more about how personality and health are connected.

# PERSONALITY AND HEALTH

Our personalities shape everything about our lives, including our health. I'm not necessarily talking about predefined personality types such as Type A or Type B, introvert or extrovert, impulsive or methodical. I'm talking about who you are as a unique individual and the way you go about living your life. When I hand a patient a treatment plan, I know that when they go home, they'll have to process it as who they are outside of the naturopathic visit and anything I've said. The patient is his or her main health guide. The more each person is willing to learn about their natural tendencies, fears, talents, strengths, weaknesses, and beliefs surrounding health and life, the more effectively they can direct their efforts toward living the way they want and supporting a healthy body and mind.

**Often, we're pressured to suppress who we are in one way or another throughout life.** Expectations placed on us, or that we place on ourselves, can make us feel like we should strive to fit in with others above everything else. We may also feel compelled to champion one side of our personalities at the expense of other sides that also need to be expressed. Unique personality can become boxed or pigeonholed. For these reasons, it's not easy to choose health.

As we talked about earlier, being healthy involves selfishness and putting yourself first. It also means risking standing out as who you are. The squashing of our unique personalities, however it comes about, suppresses the life in us and can lead to many of the chronic health issues we see today, such as low energy, hormone imbalances, mood swings, skin issues, trouble sleeping, and more. In order to truly support health, we also have to honor our personalities and who we are as individuals.

How do I investigate personality traits during a naturopathic medicine visit? One of the treatment modalities I use is called homeopathy, a unique medicinal art that connects personality to health. The homeopathic intake is comprehensive and asks not only about specific symptoms, but also the person who is experiencing the symptoms. I get to find out about a patient's common moods or emotions, food cravings, favorite time of day, activities they enjoy doing, what triggers fears and anxieties, and what he or she values in life, among other characteristics. Once I learn the "big picture" of the patient's health and personality, I can pick a specific homeopathic remedy that best treats what they are going through. Homeopathy helps spark energy and vitality, boosts the immune system, helps balance hormones, and can improve common chronic conditions that I see in practice by tapping into a person's unique personality.

---

**Challenge Questions:**

*Take a step back and try to see yourself from the outside. How would you describe yourself as an individual? What are your preferences, quirks, unique habits, morning rituals, pet peeves, food cravings, talents, challenges, and favorite things to do?*

---

Outside of the remedy itself, the homeopathic interview has real therapeutic potential. As patients talk about their personalities and approach to lifestyle in a curious and nonjudgmental way, they often begin to draw connections between who they are and their health. They learn to see that it's okay to be themselves and not label certain unique things about their personalities as "strange" or "bad." At the same time, they recognize that the "good" qualities that they do have don't necessarily have to always define who they are.

*Recognizing yourself as a unique individual plays a big part in health.* Let's look at an example of one patient who drew connections between health and personality to feel improvement in her symptoms.

A 58-year-old woman named Bridget scheduled an appointment for help with high blood pressure and anxiety. It was clear from the get-go that Bridget had experienced a lot of stress in her life that she felt had contributed to high blood pressure. Currently, she was on a hypertension medication, but she wanted help in reducing her stress naturally so she wouldn't have to rely increasingly on medication as she got older. A blood pressure reading showed that even with medication, Bridget's blood pressure was on the high end. On physical exam, her upper back and shoulder muscles were extremely tight. Bridget's whole body seemed stiff and guarded, as if she was ready to defend against some attack.

Based on Bridget's physical and emotional symptoms, exam results, and health history, I did a constitutional homeopathic intake with her. A constitutional intake is a whole-body approach to homeopathy and is better suited for chronic health issues than an acute intake. During the questionnaire,

Bridget shared that she'd had children at a very young age and raised them on her own. While she had goals to be a successful business owner in her life, raising a family single-handedly eventually wore down her efforts to do that. She had to shut down her business prematurely, which was disappointing as she'd put a lot of her hopes in it. On top of that, she and her eldest daughter didn't get along, which made Bridget feel like a failure in both her family life and in business.

Bridget shared how at age 58, she didn't feel like she'd accomplished anything she wanted in her life. She felt deficient, and the hurts that she'd experienced over time had made her a more withdrawn person than she wanted to be. The more withdrawn she felt, especially from her family, the more anxious she became about life in general. She blamed herself for the cold treatment she received from her eldest daughter. She had also given up the activities she enjoyed doing, such as reading and writing. In fact, she had a novel that she had started writing years ago that was half-finished. Bridget felt that resuming the novel again was frivolous in the face of all the problems she had with her family. She thought about these problems constantly, and when she did her stress and anxiety rose.

Bridget went home with her treatment plan, including a homeopathic remedy. At her next follow-up visit, something had shifted in Bridget. She now talked about how she had a life of her own, apart from her family, that she missed. She had gotten caught up in wanting to check off expectations, of proving herself to be a successful business owner and an excellent mother. When these things didn't go exactly as planned, Bridget felt she had failed and in a sense didn't deserve to enjoy her life. But now Bridget started to realize that she'd shouldered all the burden at the expense of her own life, and that wasn't fair to who she was. She was actually a much more passionate person than she let herself be these days, enjoying writing and studying literature. She wished she could go back to being that person instead of focusing on failed expectations from her past. The way she was living her life, she felt stress and anxiety constantly throughout her days. She wanted a change.

Talking about herself during the homeopathic intake helped Bridget think more clearly about what she wanted out of life in the present and what traits she missed about herself. She had stopped seeing herself as a unique person when she had convinced herself she was a failure in other people's eyes. She was also internalizing the criticism her eldest daughter directed toward her. Bridget wanted to return to who she really was.

Of course, it's not possible to turn back time. But as

we talked, Bridget realized that she had accomplished more than she gave herself credit for and she didn't need to redeem herself in anyone else's eyes. She owed it to herself to live her own life now that she was done raising a family, and she could shape that in any way she wanted. Over her next few follow-up visits, Bridget shared that she was writing again and enjoying the process. She had also come to accept the tension with her daughter without placing all the responsibility on herself to fix it.

Overall, she was feeling less anxious and stressed and her daily blood pressure readings were improving over time. She had decided to get a part-time job so that she could be less reliant on her children's support and live her own life. Bridget's personality also shone out more clearly during her visits, and she seemed bolder in her approach to life. She was tapping into her courage and regaining her health in the process.

The key to Bridget's improvement was not nutritional supplements, Ayurvedic herbs for stress, hypertension medications, or homeopathy. These treatments did help, but what helped the most was Bridget's openness to learn about herself and get back in touch with who she was. Stress and expectations can carry us away from being able to enjoy our personalities and life overall. When this happens, the suppression we feel can contribute to symptoms such as the high blood pressure Bridget was experiencing. Getting back in tune with ourselves, even when it feels forbidden or challenging, is an essential key in the art of health.

The way we see our health also affects how we see ourselves. There is a tendency to turn illness into a label in our society. When we focus too much on labeling what we're going through with health, we risk labeling ourselves as people too. The label can feel burdensome instead of opening up opportunities for healing and recovery. We may start to rely on that label without realizing it, feeling like the label is a big part of who we are. The next section talks about how to avoid over-labeling when it comes to health conditions.

# RIP OFF THAT HEALTH LABEL

Labels look good on canned soup, but not on people. Whether you're labeling yourself or someone is doing it to you, labels feel wrong, unfair, and confining. Health is an area where we may unfairly label ourselves without even realizing it, and the labels can get in the way of getting healthy and feeling better.

The medical world is already full of labels in the form of diagnoses. On top of that, it can be tempting to use words such as "unhealthy" or "unfit" to describe ourselves when we're not feeling our best. Those who feel uncomfortable with their weight may label themselves as "fat" when stepping on a scale. People who are experiencing emotional swings or moodiness may wonder if they're just being "hormonal." All of these words and labels can trigger feelings of inadequacy and may actually be discouraging when you're trying to improve your health.

Health happens on both physical and mental-emotional levels, so the words that we use to describe ourselves and our health do matter. It's okay to acknowledge strengths and weaknesses in health without using labels that make us feel stuck where we're at. Making healthy changes involves ups and downs, just like in life. It's a process of growth and learning, and discouraging labels don't respect the journey that it takes to get better health.

**Re-framing the words you use to describe your body and your health is just as important as the treatments that you try to improve your well-being.** Even if you're taking all the "right" steps in treatment, pushing yourself forward with punishing words and labels can block or reverse healing and recovery. A healthy mindset involves supporting yourself with the right kind of encouragement and motivation.

After a while, it's easy to become used to a health label and not question it or the presence of a health condition anymore. Frequently in my office I'll see someone who acquired the label of "diabetes" or "hypertension" from another doctor's office, only to see the condition and label as something they'll have to live with for the rest of their lives. Often after our visit, these patients realize that they don't have to enter a life sentence with that health condition and that there are real options out there that can help them feel healthier and less reliant on medications and medical labels.

In other words, just because someone has been given a diagnosis, doesn't mean that this medical-sounding word is the end of the story. Like I've described in many examples throughout this book, when two people are given the same diagnosis of "eczema," that doesn't mean they're both going through the same experience. A diagnosis is a tool that the medical community uses to classify the symptoms and conditions that arise in patients. **Unfortunately, too often a diagnosis becomes everything and prevents further investigation into how a patient can recover and feel better.**

## Challenge Question:

*Which health label, or any other kind of label, would you like to move past?*

A 55-year-old woman named Denise came to see me for help with chronic fatigue. She had received the diagnosis of "chronic fatigue syndrome" ten years ago and since then had only experienced worsening of her symptoms. Denise expressed her fears that she would be living with this diagnosis for the rest of her life. Shortly after her diagnosis, she had explored chronic fatigue chat rooms and discussion boards online for support. The longer she perused these sites, the more discouraged she became. It seemed to her that most people didn't recover from chronic fatigue syndrome, and Denise came to think that it would be her fate as well.

What scared Denise even more was that people she met in chat rooms seemed to see their lives as mostly comprised of chronic fatigue syndrome. Denise was open enough to share with me that she had started to wonder if her life would need to be all about chronic fatigue syndrome as well. While she felt tired and wanted to get better, she wasn't thrilled about the fact that her whole life might have to rotate around her diagnosis.

Denise and I talked about the effect a label can have on health. Even though the diagnosis of "chronic fatigue syndrome" could be medically useful (at times), this term did not have the right to take over her life. The more she hoisted it onto a pedestal and made it the focal point of her existence, the more it had the potential to block her health efforts and progress toward recovery. Instead, we focused on improving the specific symptoms that Denise was experiencing including trouble sleeping, chronic stress, signs of hormone imbalance, digestive upset, and weight gain. All of these symptoms fed into Denise's fatigue and without addressing them, as well as the health and strength of the whole body, Denise would remain tackling a faceless foe called "chronic fatigue syndrome."

Denise followed her treatment plan which included a homeopathic remedy, botanical medicine for relaxation and sleep, low dose natural hormone therapy, suggestions for stress relief, and a weight loss protocol.

I also encouraged Denise to pay more attention to her feelings in whatever way that made sense for her. She had a tendency to suppress so-called "negative" emotions like anger and irritation, which is something we all feel compelled to do. This suppression seemed to be trapping her energy inside along with the feelings that she didn't want to admit to having. The recommendation was simple: Denise didn't have to do anything in the moment of experiencing anger if she didn't want to. She didn't have to label herself as an "angry person" either. If a situation made her angry and her body was relaying to her signs of anger such as the digestive upset she was prone to, she could be with herself and let the body process and take care of it.

Within four months, Denise was starting to feel better and no longer felt like the words "chronic fatigue syndrome" ruled her life. It was strange, she described, that once she had gotten diagnosed with the condition, she'd almost felt like it was her duty to bear it. She had never thought that was fair, but the way that people talked about chronic fatigue syndrome she had assumed it was inevitable. Now that she felt more in charge of her health, Denise realized that a real connection with her body and her emotions was the key to getting better rather than an overemphasis on a diagnostic label.

Whether it's a medical diagnosis or a self-applied health label, it's helpful to have a suspicious and bit of a rebellious attitude when these words pop up and start ruling the mind. Many health labels have the ability to stir up a lot of needless fear surrounding recovery and healing, and at the end of the day they're just words. Some of them may offer a means of classification or path of treatment, but *they don't necessarily have to determine how we feel or our potential to get better.* If you're living with a pesky and domineering health label, time to rip it off! It may hurt in the moment, but it's healthier for the long-term and will help unleash your innate healing ability.

Denise's experience with low energy and chronic fatigue is a common issue today, without many avenues for real and effective treatment. So many people feel tired day in and day out, unable to pull together the energy they need to live life in a satisfying way. Unfortunately, the symptom of fatigue can easily become a cycle. It often leads to lack of motivation, lethargy, and stagnation. Then the inactivity that results from a low mental and physical spark promotes even more fatigue. Where is there an end in sight?

In the next section, we'll delve deeper into the topic of fatigue. It's a very broad subject and traditionally, the approach for lifting fatigue centers around things like diet, exercise, sleep, and keeping a positive attitude. We'll look at it through a different lens altogether.

# DOCTOR, WHY AM I SO TIRED?

Fatigue is such a common symptom in society, and yet it's so often that the approach to treating fatigue has become garbled or even completely ignored. Again, the thoughts that people spring to for increasing energy mostly extend *outside of themselves.* "Should I do yoga? My friend tried acupuncture, and that helped her. What about taking a multivitamin? Maybe I should jog more. Perhaps I should try and be happier and more upbeat. I bet it's time for me to go gluten-free. What is that supplement everyone's talking about that helps increase energy?"

Energy is the essential currency of life, and at every age our bodies have the ability to tap into it. Yet more and more, this innate energy feels out of reach for most people. Visiting a healthcare provider doesn't always help in this department. Frequently these days, we're visiting physicians who themselves are feeling tired and overwhelmed, who can't fathom helping someone else with the same problem. For the sake of time and business, doctors are inclined to seek and arrive at a diagnosis so they can send us on our way. The diagnosis isn't usually that helpful in guiding us on how to increase energy in our lives. If it were, conditions like chronic fatigue syndrome wouldn't be so common and difficult to treat.

Even though it may seem like you have to find the perfect thing "to take" in order to increase energy, the treatment is not where energy comes from. First we have to take a look at three important dynamics of energy that we all naturally go through:

1) Energy *entering* the body
2) Energy *leaving* the body
3) Energy *stuck* in the body

The amount of energy that is coming in, draining out, and feeling stuck holds many clues to how we feel overall. When you investigate these three dynamics, it's important to look beyond just your diet, exercise, and sleep routines. You have to look at yourself and how you live your life. What you find may surprise you, and that surprise can be the very thing that steers you in the right direction toward getting energy back for yourself. Start by asking yourself these three key questions about energy:

---

## Challenge Questions:

*1) Where is there a shortage of energy flowing in?*

*2) Which factors in life are draining your energy?*

*3) How is existing energy getting stuck?*

---

First, you can look at where there is a shortage of energy coming into your life. For a ball to roll on the ground with energy, it needs that initial push in the right direction. It takes energy to make energy. Similarly as human beings, *we need to connect with things in life that feed the energy we have inside and help it to move forward.* If you're constantly dreading the work or activities you do on a daily basis, they're not going to feed your energy. In fact, they're more likely to drain you.

To some extent, you may not have a choice in what you do for work or other responsibilities. That's okay, everyone has some limitations and restraints surrounding what they do. The key is to learn to accept the limitations that you have to deal with and to still connect with what sparks energy in your life. You owe it to yourself to bring energy into your days from things that you enjoy.

**Here's an experiment:** Pick one activity that you find fun, interesting, and engaging. Before doing this activity, look briefly in the mirror at your eyes and expression. Then go spend 20-30 minutes (or longer, if you want) on your choice of activity. Afterward, go look in the mirror. Do you notice a difference in your overall look? Does the mirror reflect back a more refreshed and rejuvenated you? If so, you just brought more energy into your life by using your existing energy. The key is, you used energy in a way that sparked your interest and excitement. It's like that saying, you have to spend money to make money. Whether you make money back or lose it depends on what you spend it on, and it is the same with energy.

As we talked about in earlier sections, resting and relaxing is a key component to health, and it is also another way to refuel your energy. As much as we feel spurred on to be superhuman and go go go, the body can't go nonstop without desiring some rest too. During rest, we help our bodies recover from both physical and mental stress. The organs and muscles get to rest, and the mind gets to relax. During this process, energy gets restored too. While you might feel guilty about resting and relaxing (many people do), you'll probably notice afterward that you're ready to go again—but with a healthier approach than if you'd driven yourself without rest. In addition to the obvious sleeping or napping, think of some low-key activities you enjoy that are relaxing for you.

Next, think about energy that is being drained. Common energy drains can come from the outside, but many of them are rooted inside too. Some of them we talked about such as the pressure to be perfect, the drive to be there for others more than for yourself, and the need for control. When you look at energy drains, the focus is not on fixing them on the spot. The very act of trying to fix ourselves can be a huge drain of energy. Instead, try and be honest about the tendencies that exist so that you can work with them and experiment with new approaches too.

For example, if you find that you're always tired after socializing, even if it's just for lunch, explore why this might be happening. Are you trying too hard to please or impress your friends? Are you giving a lot of energy away without feeling much reciprocation? Is the need to fit in with friends making it challenging to actually have fun while you're there with them? Thinking through these questions might make you feel vulnerable, but that's okay. That was just one example—everyone goes through experiences like these. But not everyone looks at them honestly, and that's where you can try a different approach.

As we talked about earlier, being too hard on yourself can also be a big drain of energy. **Are you placing pressures and expectations on your shoulders that are too heavy to carry around day after day?** Take a look at these imposed burdens and ask yourself honestly whether they're actually helping you get what you want in life. What you may find is that they're simply bringing about feelings of deficiency and disappointment that you don't need in your life and that may be draining loads of energy.

Finally, it's important to look at where energy might be getting stuck in your body and in your life. Energy can get stuck for many reasons, and we have already discussed one of the main culprits: suppressed emotions. When we're ignoring what's going on underneath the surface, these feelings fester and get buried deeper. We can convince ourselves at that point that the feelings aren't affecting our lives and that we're "over them." The body is smarter than that, however. Our suppressed emotions continue to linger inside and trap our energy in there with them. You may feel low energy and assume that you just don't have enough in the tank. The opposite may be true. You might have loads of energy inside that is just tangled with stuck or suppressed emotions that haven't had a chance to express themselves yet.

In the case of stuck emotions and energy, **it can**

**be helpful to learn to talk to yourself.** What does this mean? Talking to yourself is not a sign that you're going crazy. It's a healthy habit that can free up energy by allowing stuck emotions to flow. Imagine how you would talk to someone you know or a kid who's going through a challenging situation. For example, if you see a kid getting picked on, would you tell him or her not to feel angry? Or would you instead talk with them about how they're feeling and be supportive and encouraging? You would probably want the kid to know that they don't deserve that kind of treatment and that it's not revealing some horrible truth about them.

Often, we're much more supportive to others than we are to ourselves. You can try talking to yourself in the caring way that you might use to talk to someone else. By showing yourself some care rather than blame, disappointment, and anger for having certain feelings, those emotions can feel safer to exist in your life. If the feelings can exist more openly, they are less likely to get trapped inside along with your energy, leading to fatigue.

Learning to talk to yourself isn't always easy in a world where we're constantly surrounded by the voices of others. Living in society today, we're not openly encouraged to care about ourselves and this can lead us to talk to ourselves in unsupportive ways. If you're not used to talking to yourself in a caring way, it may seem weird at first, but give it a try. You may even find sometimes that you're actually turning to yourself first as a confidant before you decide to talk to someone else. And one more reminder—the focus is not on fixing your feelings in any way. The key is to let them exist, because they're going to anyway, either openly or entrapped in the body.

In addition to suppressed emotions, it can also be helpful to look at life in general and see where you might feel in a rut. Ruts come up in life for all of us. They may be related to our careers, family, social lives, dreams, or health. Rather than the balance and stability that can come from routines that are enjoyable, ruts can feel like the "same old,"—as if nothing is changing in the direction that we want. Again, we may have energy inside that can be used, but we can end up feeling like we're running on empty instead. The rut can seep into health as well. If you feel like life has gotten into a rut, you can look for areas in which to free up your energy toward something new that can give you energy back, like we talked about earlier in terms of energy influx.

When patients come to see me for low energy and chronic fatigue, I almost always work on balancing hormones, restoring the adrenal glands, promoting quality sleep, and supporting the immune system. At the same time, we also explore the three different facets of energy that I just talked about. When patients get familiar with ways in which their energy is draining, not replenishing, or getting stuck, they have powerful tools with which to help their treatments work even better. They also start to experiment with different approaches to energy use that can leave them feeling less tired in the future. Many of my patients may need medicine such as a natural sleep aid or adrenal support at first, but by paying attention to their energy patterns, they often start to support energy levels for the long-term and can decrease or discontinue the supplements.

The take home message of this section? **Your energy is yours!** It's easy to forget that. We get in the habit of sending our energy outward and then we end up with very little left for ourselves. If you want energy for yourself, you have to direct it toward yourself. Often, you have to reprioritize in life first in order to get that energy back. Remember, it's okay to be selfish in the art of health. After all, didn't Michaelangelo need to be selfish when he painted the Sistine Chapel? In the same way, putting yourself first is essential toward being the artist of your own health.

# HEALTH IS AN ART

True health takes courage.

If health could be sold in a bottle, it already would be by now. Despite the temptation to seek out miracle cures, our bodies and minds tell us in so many ways that just isn't the way things work. The body itself contains the greatest pharmacy of medicine that nature can make and if you can tap into that resource, you can take full advantage of your innate potential for health and healing. How do you do it? It takes listening to yourself, patience, practice, and not seeking quick fixes or magic solutions.

In this book, I talk about the many different shades of color that make up health. Health is not black and white like the text in a medical book—instead it's a colorful work of art. As you practice health as an art form, you'll develop your painter's palette more and more toward long-term health and vitality. Your health is unique to you and you are your most powerful tool in supporting it.

**The truth is, there is no medicine you can take**

**that will replace what you can do for your own health.** Different forms of medicine can act like a bridge that helps you get from where you are to where you want to go. But the bridge can't move you there directly, only you can do that for yourself. Otherwise, you end up with something that "talks the talk" of health instead of really feeling like health. We don't want health for the purpose of jotting it down on our resumes—we want health so we can feel it at our core and apply that energy throughout our lives. Health really is wealth when it comes down to it.

I can't emphasize enough how important it is to listen to yourself, not just in matters of health, but in life in general. The voice of the individual can become marginalized without us realizing it's happening. Health is blocked when we're not able to listen to our unique voices and to get in touch with what really matters to each of us. Don't let other people be the judge of who you are and what you're capable of. It's easier said than done, we all go through the similar dilemma of worrying about what others think about us. But regardless of how challenging it is to get back to your own voice and unique personality, it's worth it. Who you are is connected to your life force, which is what forms the backbone of your health.

Remember on your journey of health that you can do it, that you deserve it, and that it's already in you.

Regardless of what age you are or what your circumstances are in life, you have a right to your energy and your health. You don't have to sacrifice it for the world around you. Your body sends you messages that are like valuable clues toward health. Pay attention to what your body is saying to you, even if those around you don't find this to be important in their own lives.

**Remember to be open to learning as you go, and don't be too hard on yourself.** If you really want to get in touch with your health, you'll learn a lot about yourself and your body in the process. It's not always a comfortable feeling to admit that you don't have it all put together since there is a lot of pressure to appear that way today. But the very act of admitting to yourself that you're not perfect starts to open the door toward better health.

Finally, if you're able to see health as an art, you can have fun with it and enjoy the process too. When we entrust external sources as having all the answers about health, it introduces a lot of fear and anxiety into our lives. We don't feel like we're grabbing the reigns of our health potential and instead we're swayed by what this person or that expert says. Meanwhile, we ignore what our bodies are telling us in the moment.

Connecting to health in your own way allows you to enjoy the process of getting healthy and helps lift away fear-based approaches to the subject. It also helps you feel more in charge of your own unique health potential. Beginning to develop and trust this connection is key in your journey toward a healthier life.

Who knows best about your health? It's *you*.

# ABOUT THE AUTHOR

Aarti Patel is a naturopathic medical doctor who practices in the Bay Area, where she resides with her family. She received her doctorate in naturopathic medicine from the nation's leading program at Bastyr University. Dr. Patel is a firm believer that the journey towards health for each person involves exploring the big picture of symptoms and lifestyle imbalances. She also believes the best medicines are the ones that resonate with an individual's lifestyle and create space for natural healing.

Lightning Source UK Ltd.
Milton Keynes UK
UKHW021839081120
373036UK00017B/558